MICRO-YOGA FOR BUSY MOMS

Become a calm and fit mom with quick yoga routines

ZUZANA KOSORINOVA

To Dominik, Sam and David

Contents

Introduction

It was one day in May 2020 during the first national lock-down of the pandemic that hit the whole world and changed the way of life we had taken for granted. Because kindergartens and workplaces were closed, I was at home with my new-born son, my pre-schooler, and my husband. I was waking up many times at night to nurse the baby, entertaining my older son during the day, while cooking meals, cleaning the house, and looking after all the other household issues. I could not see my grandparent or friends, and I could not go out to any places to decompress. That day, with tears in my eyes, I thought to myself: "I lost it completely today." I yelled at my son, I was irritated at my husband, and I was too tired to be calming the baby. I was overwhelmed and exhausted, on the brink of a burnout. I could not continue like this. Something needed to change.

I needed to bring self-care back into my day. To check in with myself; to nourish and recharge my batteries. To be able to go on without losing my sanity and be able to take care of my family. I realized that I needed an activity to allow me to have some alone time. But how to find the space and the time? I was stuck at home, and I did not have time for a two-hour break. All the typical personal care providers such as salons and fitness centres were closed. I needed something quick that would benefit my body and mind, something I could do at home and that did not require a lot of resources.

I stopped crying. I saw my old yoga mat in the corner. I had not used it for some time. I had forgotten how much I loved doing yoga and how good it felt afterwards. It had not been used much in later stages of my pregnancy and after childbirth. Now I felt ready. I stepped on it, still a bit upset, and started to do some simple stretches. After a short while, I felt not only rejuvenated but also calmer. I took a deep breath in and out. I could return to my family, having the energy to care for them once again.

After some time of this kind of short practice, I realized I was onto something. These Micro-yoga breaks were vital not only for my physical strength, but also my mental wellbeing, and my productivity. I have become re-energized and calmer as a mom and a partner. Of course, I am still sometimes tired and lose my temper from time to time. I know now what my support system is and what I can do to take care of myself and improve my wellbeing.

If you are a mom with one or more kids, you are juggling many roles in your life. You do not have time to add anything extra to your day, even if it is supposed to be for your own good. You wish you had more time for yourself, for your own personal care, but the hours of the day do not add up. You are exhausted, stressed and always on-the-go. You are sleep-deprived and your back hurts. You are often on high alert. And you are frustrated that you cannot change this.

What if I told you that you can still do something nice for yourself that will bring you huge benefits over time? You can find the time for yourself as a super busy parent, and it does not require any special resources. It will not cost you anything and it requires only five minutes a day of your undivided attention and time. After experiencing the great effects of yoga rituals in my self-care journey, I decided that I wanted to share these routines and rituals with others who might find this useful. I wish for every mom to get to know the self-care routine that works for them; even when we are extremely busy with not much spare time.

Just as a side note, if you have any caring responsibilities, you can certainly try the yoga routines described in this book. Yoga is inclusive and suitable for everyone. Most of the routines are designed for all busy parents; only a certain part is particularly focused on the postnatal yoga for new moms. I primarily dedicated this book to moms because given my experience, moms tend to put their wellbeing on the backburner. Therefore, this Micro-yoga can be a great solution for them.

In this book, I will teach Micro-yoga routines I have developed that will provide you with a wonderful pathway to your own self-care, tending both to your body and mind. Surely this is something you want so you can take care of yourself, your family and other responsibilities.

You might argue that yoga is mostly done in studios by flexible people in nice yoga pants for at least an hour. What if all these assumptions about yoga might not be correct? It is a practice that is available to everyone regardless of their fitness level and it can be done anywhere even for just a few minutes per day. And you can wear anything comfortable. Moreover, it still counts as a proper practice that might be the beginning of your lifelong yoga journey.

Now imagine that you have given this a try and, in the beginning, set up an undisturbed five minutes a day for your body and mind. After some time of regular practice, you might start to see differences in how you look and feel. Yoga is proven to have a lot of physical, mental, and emotional benefits. Yoga can help with building physical strength and flexibility, decreasing stress, lowering anxiety, promoting better sleep, improving mood, and lowering fatigue. It can aid in increasing your overall wellbeing (Link, 2017). You can become a stronger, calmer, and less anxious parent and partner. And that is what we all want. You will also become someone who has a new identity – being someone who puts priority in her self-care.

In this book, I will show you routines you can easily do every day, no matter how much energy you have. First, I will look at the necessary foundations for every self-care ritual – finding the time, the space, and the supporting mechanisms to make it happen. After that, I will look at the guiding principles of all yoga routines that should be taken into consideration when beginning with yoga. I will also provide a quick overview of the yoga styles that have influenced the Micro-yoga practices in this book to describe the basic differences.

I will provide you with simple dynamic, as well as gentle Micro-yoga sequences that can be done in about five minutes per day. All the routines are designed to be accessible to people of all fitness levels, even for complete beginners. I will show you the routines step by step, so you are able to understand the entire sequence. I have divided the routines so that you will know where to begin, what to learn as the first simple routine and how to build on your practice once you have become comfortable with your first Micro-yoga practice.

After learning your first Micro-yoga sequence and becoming familiar with it, I will show you some energizing and calming routines. You can incorporate these routines into your practice depending on how you feel and what kind of practice you need. After reviewing the physical practices, I will introduce relaxation and breathing techniques that can nicely complement your physical practice and are suitable for those days when you feel low on energy.

After becoming familiar with yoga on the mat, I will introduce you to the practice off the mat and show you that Micro-yoga can be done almost anywhere - be it at work, in the park, during your commute or even in bed. These quick routines can be your go-to selection when you wish to practice, but you might not have a mat with you. After reading this book, you will have a selection of routines and tools that you can start to incorporate into your daily personal care and see the benefits of this regular practice for yourself.

My journey with yoga started more than 15 years ago, and since then yoga has become a substantial part of my life. First, I have practiced in studios during my university studies, and later I knew I wanted to move my practice to a new level. Therefore, I have attended a yoga teacher training and became a yoga instructor to be able to share the magic of yoga with others. Since 2015, I have been teaching yoga in fitness centres, corporations, in the local community, as well as private online classes. I have completed various yoga certifications such as yoga for pregnant women, face yoga, and hatha yoga.

Yoga has also been an active part of my life since becoming a mom. Yoga has accompanied me during both of my pregnancies, after giving birth, during my maternity leave and after returning to work. Before and during motherhood, it has never failed to give me physical strength, flexibility, balance, peace of mind and other benefits.

The reason for writing this book is that I have experienced first-hand that Micro-yoga practice can work wonders for busy moms. And I wanted to share it with others who might be in a similar situation. I wanted all moms to be able to claim at least a couple minutes per day for themselves to do something beneficial for their body and mind. Of course, five minutes of yoga per day for your personal care might be just a beginning. Slowly, day by day, you might be able and eager to do a bit more and want to spend more time with yourself looking after your body and mind.

It is good to first understand what this book can offer and what it cannot. This book will not carve out time for your personal care. However, it will provide you with tips on how to find time for your quick me-time and who to involve to make it happen. Moreover, it will equip you with simple routines based on yoga tradition. These sequences will be ready for you whenever you have a couple of minutes to spare at home or elsewhere. And I can guarantee that even five minutes a day regularly doing something great for your body and mind can have a profound effect. Micro-yoga practice might not make your back pain go fully away, it might not make you lose weight, and it might not release all the stress you might have. The primary goal of the Micro-yoga practice taught in this book is to find quality time for yourself every day. It is still possible though that over time this consistent practice will lead you to more toned body, calmer mind and feeling more at ease.

If all of this sounds intriguing, welcome aboard on your new Micro-yoga journey. I promise it will be worth it. But first, let us look at how moms got to where we are with our personal care and how Micro-yoga can help us with it.

Self-care for Moms

When we become moms, self-care is often regarded as the lowest priority. And it should not be like that. When we nourish ourselves, we can nourish those around us and those we care for.

The benefits of finding time for ourselves and our own wellbeing are endless. Benefits of self-care are known for decades and have been written about in numerous studies; better health and fitness, more productivity, more life satisfaction as well as better relationships with your family and partner (BMIHealthcare, 2021). Other benefits of self-care include lowering stress levels and frustrations, being better partners with more energy and more patient parents (Christina M Godfrey, 2010). It also helps to maintain our sense of self-worth. Taking care of ourselves will help us remember our interests and our identity beyond motherhood. It also sets a good example for children and teaches them to value health and well-being.

On the other hand, when we neglect our self-care, we risk caregiver burnout which is created by physical, emotional, and mental exhaustion and leads to more physical sickness, or mental health issues (Shortsleeve, 2019). When we do not take care of ourselves on a regular basis, it can affect our physical condition, resulting in a weaker immune system and high blood pressure. It can also affect our mental health, leading to a higher risk of depression and anxiety.

Again, this does not happen overnight, but slowly day by day, when we forget to take time aside to connect with ourselves to care for our body and mind. According to the author of Atomic Habits, James Clear, it is when we repeat tiny errors, it leads to toxic results. The accumulation of many small missteps eventually leads to a big problem (Clear, 2018).

Intuitively, we know all of this but as busy moms, it can be hard to find time for ourselves. In our hectic world, according to research, moms have only 17 minutes for themselves a day (Kirkova, 2014). In general, parents get less than an hour a day of me-time (Schmall, 2018). Of course, this is due to the reality of modern life and all the roles we have. Being a mom often means being the coach, the taxi-driver, the mentor, the professional worker, the nanny, the cleaner, the cook, and many other roles all at the same time. As a result, we have only a limited amount of time for activities that promote our own wellbeing.

We tend to look after everyone else. We have chores, work and caring responsibilities, and our schedules are packed. We feel the need to do everything before we allow ourselves to unwind and rest. And we repeat the cycle every day until our body, our mind or something else sends us a strong signal that we need to put ourselves on the priority list again.

I have certainly been this way all my life until I had my second child. I felt that I need to run all the errands, do all the chores, and have all my work to-do list done before I could sit down and relax. What usually happened was that as soon as I had a vacation or a break from work or family, I became ill. Also, I felt quite irritable because I was running on low fuel and had not recharged my batteries. And secretly I felt frustrated that I do not have even five minutes completely for myself. I understood only after my second child was born and I was almost burnt out that it is not selfish to take care of yourself – I need to have my resources full so I can give and care for the entire family. After taking at least five minutes for myself every day and being strict about that, I have found wonderful benefits; acting calmer towards my kids, being kind to my husband and generally happier and content.

Thus, self-care is not about the great interventions that you do only a couple times a month like going for a massage or going for a swim. Of course, those are all fine activities, but they would not be sufficient on their own. As a mom of two young boys, I understand very well that parents do not often have two hours for their own hobbies.

Rather, it is the small, daily practices that will define how you feel in the long run. Self-care activities can be built into our days no matter how busy we are and what type of jobs and other responsibilities we hold. And it is these small activities that have value in our lives and make all the difference in the long term.

We need to start looking at self-care as an investment into our own wellbeing and into better care for our families. By taking the time to check in each day with the body and mind, we connect with our own source of wellbeing. This is a highly effective act of self-love.

Therefore, personal care is not a luxury but rather a necessity for us and our families. We might already feel so overwhelmed with all the duties and other activities that we do not want to add anything else to our to-do list. Yet, taking care of yourself does not have to be time consuming. The way forward is thus to inject small doses of personal time into our days. Do something beneficial for your body and mind for five minutes at a time. This is a great way to start. Of course, this is only the beginning and over time you will find it worthwhile to further increase your time devoted to self-care. This book will teach you your first Micro-yoga self-care strategies to get started; both on the mat and off the mat.

Before we look at the Micro-yoga routines, you might be asking yourself: Why exactly should you choose Micro-yoga for the daily go-to personal care ritual? What benefits can it have and how can you manage it?

Why Micro-yoga for Moms?

The foundation of yoga is harmony between the body and mind. Yoga allows us to concentrate fully on the present moment and dedicate full attention to ourselves, to our bodies and minds. This concentration allows us to let go of other worries we have, at least for a while. Because of this, I have chosen yoga as my primary self-care tool as a mom.

In this book, I will introduce techniques and routines that are accessible for all moms and can be done almost anywhere in a minimum amount of time.

Here are ten reasons why yoga is a great self-care tool for moms. Research shows these benefits of regular yoga practice for the physical and mental health:

1. Increasing flexibility.
2. Building physical strength and toning muscles.
3. Balancing metabolism.
4. Detoxifying the body.
5. Lowering blood pressure.
6. Improving digestion.
7. Strengthening immunity.
8. Improving sleep.
9. Aiding our parasympathetic nervous system and helping the mental state.
10. Releasing anxiety and helping with depression (Woodyard, 2011).

Moreover, yoga can help with a lot of common mom's issues such as: lack of sleep, lower energy, stress, negative emotions, fluctuating hormones, a weakened immune system, issues with body confidence and difficulties with relationships (Kaur, 2016). From my personal experience, after doing a regular yoga practice at home, I started to sleep better, have better flexibility, balance, and muscle strength, and I have become less anxious and more peaceful. With consistent Micro-yoga practice, I have become a more energized mom and a happier partner.

Study after study has shown that if we want to adopt a new habit or change our behaviour in some way, we need to design the new routine to be as effortless as possible (Clear, 2018). If we want to rely on our stamina and willpower, we will not succeed, and the new routine will not survive in our daily life. That is why my Micro-yoga routines are designed to be as easy as possible and are all accessible for complete beginners.

Starting with something new on a super easy level is a powerful strategy because once we have started doing the right thing and we are successful in achieving this on a regular basis, it boosts our motivation to continue (Clear, 2018). I always feel accomplished when I achieve even a short yoga routine in a day because I have spent at least some time mindfully engaging with myself.

Research shows that when you are starting with something new, it is key to start with a simple routine so you will stick with it even when the conditions are not ideal (Clear, 2018). However, when the new habit has been established it is important to continue to advance in small ways to keep the motivation levels up. So perhaps once we can do Micro-yoga for five minutes a day, we can extend that to ten or fifteen minutes to increase the feel-good factor.

Doing yoga related self-care activities for a few minutes a day is going to be more beneficial than a long workout once every other week or pampering with an occasional massage. It is a journey where we engage with ourselves on a regular basis and make a daily decision to prioritize our own wellbeing. This then allows us to be able to care for others and manage other duties. According to Dr Chatterjee, it is the daily habits that will have the most fundamental effect on our lives (Chatterjee, 2019). The reason is that "Habits are the compound interest of self-improvement. A small habit—when repeated consistently—grows into something significant (Clear, 2018)."

We sometimes tend to believe that our busy schedule prevents us from our own self-care and any other beneficial exercise. However, having a tight schedule and other responsibilities can help us develop qualities that are necessary for a continuous yoga practice and other self-care routines. These typical mom skills include flexibility, stamina, and patience.

Flexibility requires us to be able to adapt very quickly to the changing needs of our children and juggle different priorities at the same time. Children's needs are always changing, and we need to be responsive and ready to change according to them. Mental flexibility means that we will be ready to creatively integrate yoga and other self-care practices into our already busy agenda. Also, we will be able to adjust our self-care practice, considering our energy, how we feel, and what our family needs.

We also need to have a lot of stamina to be able to keep up with a job, look after our family and household, and other responsibilities. If we have the strength to do all that, then we can practice Micro-yoga. When we begin this new habit with resilience and endurance, we will not give up on the practice, even when life gets in the way.

Finally, patience is considered a profound quality of moms. Even when we feel we do not have it and we are not patient enough, we are certainly building it throughout the entire motherhood. For instance, just remind yourself how you can patiently respond to a crying new-born, a persistent toddler trying to reach for something they cannot have or constant questions of your pre-schooler – you see how much patience that requires. This quality will enable you to be patient on your new Micro-yoga journey. Patience is necessary when you need to listen to your body to understand what it needs on a particular day and not push yourself over your limit. Only patient practice brings long-term results.

I believe that any mom can benefit from regularly doing yoga for five minutes a day. Dedicating five minutes during the day to your self-care is better than not doing anything at all and it will have profound benefits when done regularly. And who knows, maybe some days you might want to extend your practice to longer time if you can. The key thing is that slowly, day by day, you will become a parent and a partner who value your self-care and take care of your body and mind. Your personal care will not be just a phrase, but you will value it and prioritize it daily. After a consistent practice for at least a few weeks, it will be visible that Micro-yoga is beneficial for you, your wellbeing, and your relationships.

Before introducing the Micro-yoga routines, we will look at the required space, time, support, and the right mindset. These are all necessary foundations for any new yoga self-care routine.

Creating "Mom's Sanctuary"

Creating our own sanctuary at home means finding a space that we can claim as our own; where we can be undisturbed for at least five minutes per day. The mom's sanctuary is a safe space where we can come even just for a short time and wind down, relax, or do a refreshing activity. A sanctuary can be a favourite armchair, a kitchen table with a cup of tea and a magazine, or a little corner at home to practice our hobbies.

The mom's sanctuary is quite an important space in triggering the activity connected with this place in the mind. According to research, when we want to create a new routine, we need to make our environment and our system as supportive of the new habit as possible. The right environment makes our new habits more likely to be achievable (Clear, 2018).

At my home, this type of sanctuary is my yoga mat. It can change places, sometimes being taken from our bedroom to the living room. Wherever it is, it symbolizes me coming home to myself; to reconnect and nourish my body and soul. Being stored in a visible spot also acts as a trigger to get on it every single day, even if it means just lying down for a quick relaxation.

Before starting the yoga routine, the task for you is to find a small space in your home where you can dedicate the time for your new self-care habit. It does not require much – you just need a space where you will not be disturbed for a short while and where you have a yoga mat (or a carpet can work just as well). You can also decorate it with a candle or play some gentle music when you step on the mat, but this is up to you.

Once you have this space dedicated to your practice, your motivation will go up and you are almost ready to go.

After you have set up a space for your new personal care practice, you should look for the right time that you can dedicate to this activity and think about the support and mindset you will need to make it stick.

Scheduling "Me-time" and Establishing the Right Mindset

Another significant part of making your new self-care routine stick is to carve out a special time for yourself, even if it is only a few minutes for this activity each day.

Involvement of your partner, nanny or any other child-care support who can look after the kids while you are trying something new can prove to be a great help. Before the start, it is worthwhile to involve a partner into this schedule if possible. It is beneficial if you explain that you would like to do something good for your body and mind every day to be able to have more energy for all your other responsibilities. I have done this when I wanted to go back to doing yoga after having my second child. I felt I needed some time for myself and my body each day. Therefore, I asked my husband to do the bath-time with my older son and after I put down my younger baby into his crib at bedtime, I had time to do my quick routine every day.

Be clear about what time is best for you to have a yoga practice. Once you have decided which time works best for you, then go and discuss this with your partner or someone who you would like to involve helping you. After it is set in stone that they will look after the kids at the time (if this is needed at that specific time), you will be less likely to be disturbed and have more motivation to go ahead with your routine.

Of course, I understand that everybody's schedule is different and not everyone has available childcare support. I have offered my personal tip that works in my life. I understand this won't be suitable for all moms. What I would recommend to everyone is trying to work out how to fit this self-care routine into your day. For instance, scheduling it in your calendar, setting up a reminder into your phone, or planning these yoga breaks a week in advance might be helpful when you have a more irregular week flow or little support available.

The best time to schedule your mini-me breaks is when you know you will not forget about them. That means placing them into your daily routine when it works for you. This will be different for everyone. First thing in the morning before everyone gets up works for some moms, for others it is during their lunch break or during the child's nap, or at the end of the day when children are tucked in bed. Think about what time could work best for you before you start the routine. Once this self-care habit has been established, you can also add more ad-hoc Micro-yoga slots throughout the day. When starting out though, it is key to have the time and the place set in stone.

It is also crucial to set up your mind for success in the long run. It is important to view self-care not as a luxury but as fuel to drive your engine. This fuel will enable you to care for your family each day. This mindset of putting your own self-care first should be without any sense of guilt. You need to give yourself permission to look after your body and mind first because you deserve to be cared for and to be able to refuel your energy. What can help is to remind yourself that doing something for yourself, however tiny, will boost your energy, and help you unwind. In addition, if you do something for yourself that brings you energy, and joy and a peace of mind, then you can be a happier and more attentive parent. In the end, it is a win-win situation for everyone.

After setting up the physical and mental requirements for the new habit, let us look at how we can elevate this new routine to a self-care ritual.

Creating a Self-care Ritual

Routines are repetitive actions that help us develop skills and create order and familiarity. Both routines and rituals help us define space and time by creating predictable structure, continuity, and rhythm. Rituals differ from routines because they lift us up and create excitement. They are elevated by creativity, driven by intention, and infused with meaning (Perel & Miller, 2020).

When we create a ritual out of our yoga routine, we can transform an ordinary practice into something significant. When we repeat our routine consistently and with a focused intention and personal purpose, this yoga routine transforms into a self-care ritual. Our Micro-yoga can be elevated to a ritual by the intention and by the creativity that we bring into our sacred time and by the purpose of self-love that drives this activity.

We can create a ritual out of a short exercise routine when we invite intention, creativity, and meaning into it. There might be many ways how you can invite positive intention into your yoga practice. For instance, at the beginning of every practice, I put my hands in a prayer position in front of my heart, close my eyes and inhale in deeply. While I take a deep breath, I set the intention for my practice. How to set a positive intention will be described in the next chapter.

Next, make this Micro-yoga practice special by being creative around engaging your senses. This way you will become fully present, and you will be able to enjoy the practice more. According to the author of Effortless Greg McKeown, rituals are habits with a soul (McKeown, 2021). I like to light a candle for an evening practice, play specific instrumental gentle music and spray a calming fragrance around my yoga mat. At the end, I usually close the practice by putting my hands together in front of my chest and invite gratitude into my mind. I am thankful for being able to find the time for myself and for my body being able to exercise. This way, I am creating an important ritual out of what would otherwise have been just a regular yoga exercise.

Finally, the most important part is to elevate a simple act of exercising to a self-love ritual by understanding the value of these precious minutes. The real purpose of this practice is checking in with your body and mind, spending quality time with yourself and turning inward to connect with your identity.

As you can see, it is quite easy to create a special self-care ritual for yourself out of a simple routine. Let us try to remember this when we step on the mat for the first time to invite intention, creativity and meaning into our practice.

Alongside the physical and mental foundations to create a new yoga self-care ritual, I will now introduce you to yoga's guiding principles. We should be aware of these guidelines when starting any form of yoga practice.

Micro-yoga Guidelines

There are a few general guidelines I have been following in my Micro-yoga practice that I find useful. Some of these are well-known in the yoga world, some of them I have adopted from my yoga teachers and some I have learnt during my long-term practice. When you tune in to your body and find out what works for you, you might be able to establish some of your own guidelines. Try to remember these guidelines as you come to the mat. Your practice will become easier and more meaningful.

1. MOVEMENT FOLLOWS BREATH.
    This is a widely known rule in yoga. There is a natural flow of breathing and movement. Awareness of your own breathing is a cornerstone in yoga. Breath influences how our mind and body works. Movement in yoga not only follows breath but breathing initiates the movement and there is a synchronicity between moving and breathing. That means that we move after each inhale and then again after each exhale. We let the breath be our guiding force. Try not to hold your breath but breathe in sync with the movement. This is how yoga differentiates from any other physical exercise (Ekhart, 2021). It may take you a little while to synchronize your breathing with movement and that's alright. You will get there in your own time.

2. LISTENING TO OUR BODIES AND AHIMSA (THE PRINCIPLE OF NON-VIOLENCE).
    Always listen to your body and be gentle with yourself. This is the principle of ahimsa. Ahimsa is a principle of non-violence and is based on the ancient yoga wisdom. It applies to all living creatures; including yourself and your body. Never force any yoga posture (asana) through pain. Pain is a signal from your body that you might be stretching too much and pushing too far into the pose and that your body is not ready for it. If your body gives you a signal that you need to push less, accept the range of motion and flexibility your body has. Yoga practice should never be about pain; it should bring you joy and a nice stretch. How you can get into a more intense stretch in any pose is by releasing into the pose fully with an exhale.

3. BALANCE.
    It is essential to learn to inhale - to get energy - to be able to exhale and to release energy around us. That is why self-care is so significant: it is our way to inhale. In this case, our breath shows us the two sides of the same coin. With an inhale, we breathe in the oxygen that brings the necessary nourishment of our cells and enables the energy in our bodies to circulate. With an exhale, we release carbon dioxide, and we prepare our body for the intake of oxygen. Inhalation is like expanding to new things, bringing in new energy, and opening to new possibilities. Exhalation is a powerful metaphor for releasing our body of anything that does not serve us anymore and giving up the things that we do not need anymore.

Balance between inhalations and exhalations can be soothing and physiologically healing, calming our nervous system, and supporting the functioning of our immune system. This is the principle of finding the balance between effort and ease (EkhartYoga, 2021).

Based on this principle, we choose the right practice for each day and our needs. Sometimes that might be a gentle restorative routine and another times, a strong dynamic flow. This principle can apply not only to our yoga practice but also to how we live our life off the mat. Understanding that we need to rest when we feel run-down and stressed. Or, on the other hand, when we need to bring a bit more action into our efforts.

4. PRACTICING CONCENTRATION.
When we concentrate on our breathing, we subsequently focus on each movement that follows. Our mind is connected to our body movement and is not wandering. It is there with us on the mat. When practising vinyasa yoga, I can experience a wonderful flow state. This practice requires me to concentrate on movement and does not allow me to think about what I need to do later or what went well or did not go so well that day. I am following my breath and movement and that enables me to enter the state of concentration.

5. INTENTION IS KEY.
What makes yoga different from many other physical exercises is intention. Intention in Sanskrit is called Sankalpa. Kalpa means vow and San means a connection with our high-

est truth. We set an intention at the beginning of our practice because we want to dedicate the practice to a quality that we want to carry for the whole duration of our practice. It should be a positive statement that we would like to emulate during our practice. We also should utilize it in our daily life off the mat. The intention is deeply personal, it should be something true to us and what we want to focus on. And it gives our practice a more profound meaning.

To set an intention is not difficult; simply focus on your breathing and tune inward. Bring your awareness to what matters to you on that day and what you would like to embody. It can be anything - just keep the statement short and positive. For instance, I am relaxed. I am flexible. I am resilient. I am full of love. I think of my intention at the end of my practice as part of my final relaxation. It is also recommended to bring it back into your mind at any point during the practice - especially during more challenging poses - as it might make your breathing through the pose a bit easier.

6. EVEN LYING ON A YOGA MAT IS A PRACTICE.
I completely agree with this statement. On a bad day, even one full and concentrated deep breath in and out counts more than a distracted practice for an hour. And even lying on a mat in a relaxation pose is a practice. The key thing is coming back to the mat every day. Relaxation is a crucial part of yoga, and we should take advantage of this. We should embrace the fact that we might not have the energy for physical practice every day, especially after challeng-

ing and busy days with kids and other responsibilities. But we can always find a couple of minutes for our favourite relaxation position. The most important thing is to keep showing up for yourself and keep checking in with your body and mind on the mat.

7. BE GRATEFUL FOR YOUR BODY AND DO NOT COMPARE YOURSELF TO OTHERS.
    Each of us has a different body, range of motion and flexibility. During yoga practice, especially with other people, this becomes very apparent. Some people are hyper-flexible and can do very advanced poses. Nowadays, in our highly competitive world, we compare ourselves to others even during yoga practice. We tend to push our bodies beyond their physical limits only to copy others in the class. This is counterproductive as it creates pain in our body and potentially even injury. Therefore, we need to follow the yoga principle of Santosha: being content with the body we have and its abilities. We should accept our bodies the way they are - and how they perform during practice - without judgement and constant comparison to others. Of course, resisting comparison is much easier during home practice, but the mindset remains the same. We should be content with and grateful for the abilities of our body and accept the range of motion it can offer. Slowly, we will build on these abilities over time.

8. SHOWING UP ON THE MAT IS THE ACCOMPLISHMENT.
    As it is often said, the first step is often the hardest. You should give

yourself a small pat on the back when you get on the mat and just manage a standing tall Mountain Pose with deep inhales and exhales. Even doing this for five minutes can bring great respite. On a bad day, accomplishing even one pose is a huge success. And perhaps the next time you manage a couple rounds of Sun Salutation yoga flow. Remembering that your yoga mat lies in the corner and stepping on it is the most important part of your practice and everything else follows.

9. YOGA CAN BE PRACTICED ANYWHERE.
    What is wonderful about yoga is that you do not need to go to the yoga studio to be able to practice. You do not need to own a super shiny yoga mat and a new pair of yoga pants. You can do yoga in your house, where you work, in the park with your kids, in a hotel room; almost anywhere. All you need is a bit of space for yourself, some comfortable clothes, and a mindset of curiosity. You can do yoga even on the carpet or a floor, and even in your pyjamas! I know this very well because when practicing in the house with kids sometimes the practice might be messy, or distracted, but I often decide to just go with it and enjoy it anyhow. Yoga is more about the mindset rather than the location.

10. ENJOY IT!
    This might be the most important guideline of all. Enjoy it. Without joy you will not be able to continue in the long run. Micro-yoga is super quick, so make sure you try to enjoy every movement and every breath. When

we enjoy something, we bring our full selves to the activity and our motivation to repeat it increases. During and after yoga, you should feel nicely stretched and relaxed; you should be able to enjoy the rest of your day even more. Once you have tried a few routines in this book, try to find at least one you enjoy best and practice it regularly.

Before stepping on the mat to learn our first micro-routine, I will provide a quick overview of the most common yoga styles which have influenced the routines in this book.

Finding the Right Yoga Style

There are many styles of yoga, so it can be quite overwhelming for a non-practitioner to choose which one to start with. In this book, I have utilized various yoga styles described below to create my Micro-yoga routines. They suit different needs moms might have on different days. I have also added some other yoga practices such as relaxation, breathing, and meditation that are usually part of all yoga styles.

Without further ado, let me introduce the main yoga styles that have influenced my practice. This overview is included to give you an idea of each style with its particular focus.

HATHA YOGA
This is the foundation of all yoga styles. It is based on an ancient system that includes the asana practice (yoga positions) and pranayama (breathing) exercises that enable peace of mind and body, preparing the body and mind for deeper meditation practice. Its overall goal is to achieve enlightenment. Today, hatha is used as a very general term to cover most of yoga classes offered. Usually, these classes will be gentle, slower and with a more relaxed pace.

VINYASA YOGA
This general term can describe many different styles of yoga which are quite dynamic and vigorous. Typically, in vinyasa yoga we see a continuous flow of yoga postures and movement synchronized with breathing. It is usually based on a flow of Sun Salutations (a sequence of yoga poses) and its variations.

POWER YOGA
This yoga style is very vigorous, physically demanding, and close to vinyasa style. It originated from a very rigorous practice of Ashtanga yoga in the United States as an attempt to make it more accessible and suitable for a Western audience. However, there is no prescribed sequence like in Ashtanga. It resembles vinyasa as it enables the yoga teacher to choose a sequence at will.

YIN YOGA
This yoga style can be gentle, and poses are held for a longer time. It is more passive in nature. This practice works more with joints than muscles and focuses on working the connective tissues in the body.

It is good to understand different yoga styles because everyone has different needs and lifestyle. Thus, it is best to choose the right type of yoga that supports your daily rhythm and lifestyle. Each mom also has a different body. Therefore, you might need to personalize your sequence once you understand the correct execution of each movement. Attention to your body will usually tell you which movement is appropriate for you, and which one is not.

Furthermore, we feel different on each day and thus we might need a different routine every day. It is good to keep this in mind. Sometimes when we feel full of energy and want to give our body a bit of a workout to promote our physical strength, it is good to follow a more dynamic yoga sequence based on the power or vinyasa yoga style. On those days when we feel really overwhelmed by our duties or stressed, it is good to include a gentler practice based on a restorative hatha or yin yoga style. Therefore, in this book I have prepared a selection of dynamic and gentle Micro-yoga routines available for every mom to choose from based on her current needs.

Having covered where my Micro-yoga practice has its influences, I will now introduce a Micro-yoga routine suitable after giving birth. Then, we will look at a standard routine that can be incorporated into your daily practice.

Micro-yoga Practice for a New Mom

After giving birth to my second son, life got much busier. I did not have time to exercise to get back in shape. And I needed to be fit to support my family and look after my sons and my husband. I quickly realized that time is limited, so I needed to be super-efficient with my exercise. Thus, I found small amounts of time for micro-doses of yoga. This Micro-yoga - as I started to call it - really transformed my body back to my old self. It brought back quality self-care to my days.

I gave birth to both my sons naturally and was fortunate to have a quick labour without major complications in both cases. Thus, my recovery was relatively quick, and I could start light exercise a couple of weeks after labour. I exercised different safe post-natal micro-sequences - about five minutes at a time, sometimes fifteen minutes when I was lucky. In a couple months' time I found remarkable results - I was on my pre-pregnancy size and felt fit again.

Every day I found at least five minutes – after I put my baby into his crib for the night. While he was dozing off and the older one was in the bath with his dad watching him, I worked out on the floor in my bedroom. I laid down a small carpet which I used as a mat for my practice. My practice consisted of full yoga breathing which is founded on the expansive belly breathing. This means concentrating the full cycle of breath into the belly. Your belly expands when you inhale and slightly contracts when you exhale.

Slowly, after the first six weeks, I felt I had more energy to start my regular ha-tha yoga practice. I adjusted this practice to include more postnatal exercises and exercises to heal belly gap - diastasis recti. I did not have such an extensive belly gap, but I still wanted to work on my core strength. It is important to strengthen stomach muscles to avoid back pain typical for moms caring for young infants and to maintain a good posture.

The results of this regular micro-practice were incredible: in just four months' time I could do the same practice as I could before my pregnancy. I was able to fit into my pre-pregnancy clothes and I felt fit and strong. I also felt calmer and more at ease. I was really enjoying my family and my motherhood.

Given my personal experience, I wholeheartedly recommend trying the post-partum Micro-yoga practice to all moms, whether with new-born baby or older kids. This specific routine will be introduced in the next chapter. You will see that finding the time for a regular practice will be beneficial to your body, as well as your mind, and will have ripple effects that will affect your life off the mat.

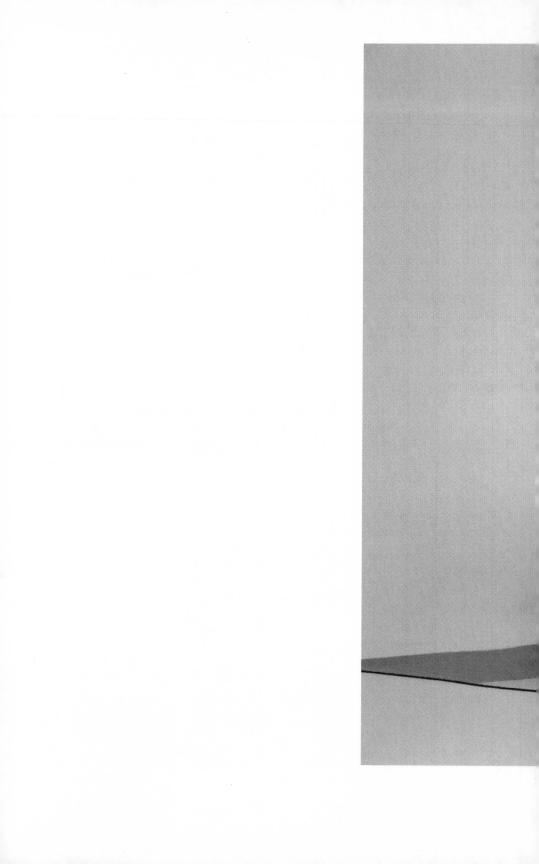

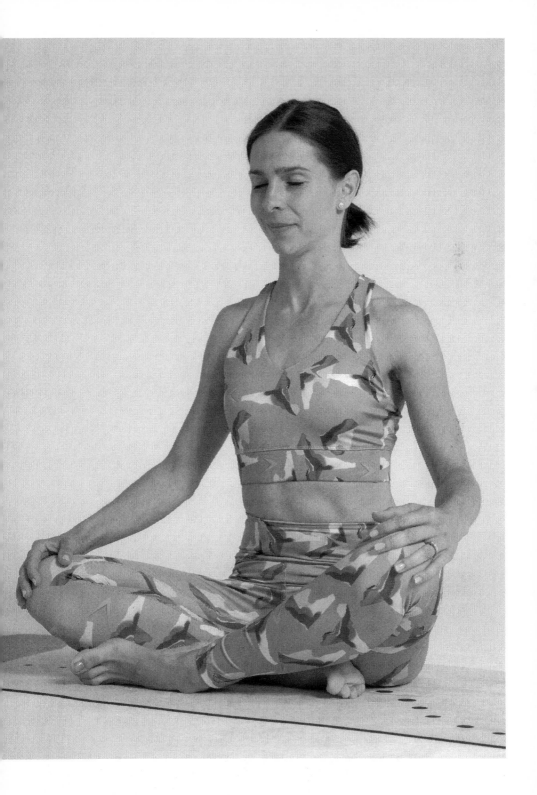

A Postpartum Micro-yoga Routine

In this part I will introduce my postpartum practice. You can also try it, even if you have not given birth lately. In general, these micro-postnatal exercises are designed for the first three months after giving birth. However, they can be still beneficial for your pelvic floor muscles after you are no longer a new mom. Even if you gave birth two years ago, introducing short pelvic floor exercises into your exercise routine might be helpful. This is useful because your pelvic muscles and tissue can weaken during pregnancy and are strained during childbirth which can lead to pelvic floor issues. Pelvic floor issues after pregnancy are usually connected with bladder control issues, pain in the pelvis area, and pain during sex. It is better to check with your doctor to ask about any issues. One thing you can do on your own as a part of your self-care routine is to start doing simple pelvic floor exercises. When done consistently, these exercises will help to strengthen your pelvic floor muscles and may help with the above-mentioned issues.

After the first three months, you can continue with the first Micro-yoga routine introduced in the next chapter. If you are not after childbirth and want to start learning the standard routines, you can skip this chapter and go onto the next one.

All exercises in this chapter have tremendous benefits when done consistently. When you find yourself exhausted after doing a few exercises or you are interrupted during this practice, don't fret. It is better to do at least a few of these exercises than doing nothing. Start slowly and listen to what your body is telling you. Be kind to yourself. The most important thing is coming back to your mat and doing any exercises regularly.

Rules to follow with these exercises:

1. Perform each move carefully and slowly.
2. Practice deep inhalation and exhalation with each move.
3. Be mindful of any tension and stop if you feel any excess pressure or any pain.
4. Always consult a doctor prior to beginning any exercise regime after giving birth.

① PELVIC FLOOR EXERCISES

These gentle pelvic floor exercises can be done as early as on the second day after giving birth if you have been cleared by your doctor. If you ever feel any discomfort or pain, stop exercising and just continue to breathe.

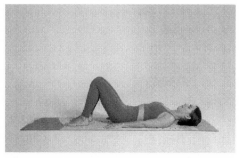

→ Lie on your back and bend your legs. Close your eyes and pull your glutes towards you. This will engage your pelvic floor muscles. These are the muscles you use when you hold your urine. Repeat 5 times.

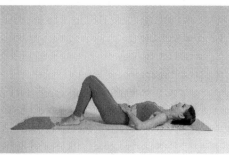

→ Lie on your back and bend your legs. Put your palms on your lower ribs. Inhale into your chest, exhale with your mouth. Repeat 5 times. Move your hands to your belly. Inhale in, expanding your belly. Exhale, pulling your belly in and lower back onto the floor, engaging your pelvic floor. Then release. Repeat 5 times.

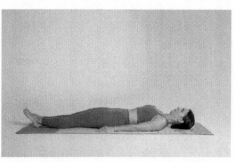

→ Lie on your back with your legs straight. Pull your knees, your thighs, and glutes together. Breathe into your chest, suck in your belly and exhale slowly. Repeat 5 times.

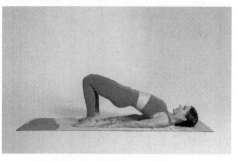

→ Stay on your back with your legs bent. Inhale into your belly as you lift your pelvis and your hips towards the ceiling until you come into the half bridge pose. Exhale and slowly move vertebra-by-vertebra back onto the mat. Repeat 3-5 times.

② MICRO-YOGA EXERCISES FOR HEALING DIASTASIS RECTI

Diastasis recti is a separation of the abdominal muscles that can happen during pregnancy when muscles make space for the growing baby. The separation can occur anywhere from the top of the midline to the bottom, or from the bottom of the breast-bone to the top of the pubic bone. In short, this gap between your right and left abdominal muscles can result in a protruding belly. Diastasis recti is not only a visual inconvenience, but it can also lead to some health issues: such as back pain, pelvic pain, and worsened trunk mobility.

It is quite easy to check if you have diastasis recti. You can easily do it when lying on your back with your knees bent and feet on the floor. Put one hand on your belly with your fingers on your midline on top of your belly button. Press your fingers down gently and bring your head up. Feel if your abdominal muscles have a gap between them that is thicker than one finger.

Certain exercises are prohibited when you are trying to treat diastasis recti, as they might exacerbate the gap. Most traditional abs exercises, such as crunches, are going to worsen this condition. Thus, it is recommended to avoid any exercise that places strain on your midline or causes your belly to bulge forward; such as plank or sit-ups.

Something that is recommended that might help with diastasis recti are exercises which strengthen the core and keep the belly pulled in; such as the ones in the sequence recommended below. These are some basic exercises that you can start with. They can be done right after delivery if you have been cleared by your doctor and you feel healthy. As soon as you feel stronger in your core, you can slowly move on to the more advanced versions or do more repetitions.

Sequence:
1. PELVIC TILTS
2. LEG SLIDES
3. SINGLE LEG LIFT
4. TOE TAPS
5. SINGLE LEG REACH

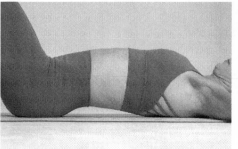 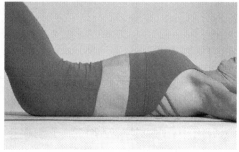

1. **PELVIC TILTS**
→ Lie on your back with your knees bent and the soles of your feet on the mat. In this neutral position, the natural curve of your lumbar spine will lift your lower back slightly off the floor.

→ Exhale and gently rock your hips toward your head. With this movement you can feel your lower back pressing into the floor. Focus on engaging your abdominal muscles. Stay here for 5 breaths and then return to the neutral position.

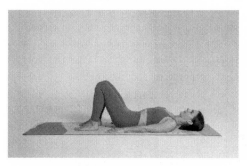 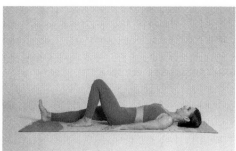

2. **LEG SLIDES**
→ Lie on your back. Keep your arms by your side and let your right leg slide slowly towards the mat and back. Make sure your heel is always touching the mat while sliding. Think about tilting your pelvis and belly in as you slide. Repeat 10 times with each leg.

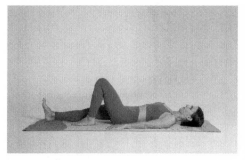

3. **SINGLE LEG LIFT**
→ Lie on your back on the mat: your left foot on the ground, left knee bent, and your right leg extended. Place your hands by your side.
→ Inhale. With an exhale, slowly raise your extended leg toward the ceiling until it reaches a 45-degree angle to the floor. Keep your lower back flat on the mat during the entire lift. Keep the right knee straight. Pull your navel in and toward your spine for core engagement.
→ Inhale as you slowly return the leg down. Repeat 10 times, then switch sides.

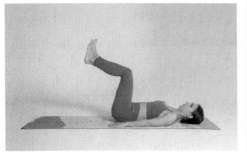 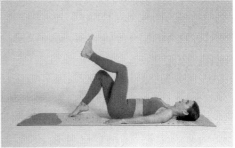

4. TOE TAPS
→ Lie flat on your back, bring your legs to a Tabletop position with your knees directly over your hips. Make sure you do not arch your back or tuck your pelvis.
→ Inhale into your ribcage and exhale as you tap your right foot on the floor, drawing in your core.
→ Inhale as you return to neutral. Perform 10 times on each side.

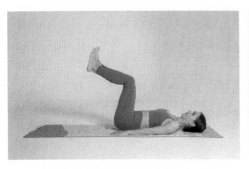 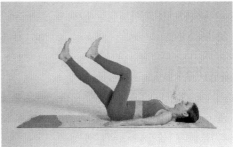

5. SINGLE LEG REACH
→ Lie on your back. Begin in Tabletop position and keep your pelvis still. As you exhale, extend your right leg as if trying to reach the opposite wall.
→ Inhale as you return to neutral.
→ Repeat 10 times on each side.

In the next chapter, we will look at one standard energizing routine and one calming routine that you can do every day. You can alternate between them based on the energy level you have that day.

Standard Energizing Micro-yoga Routine

You have decided to do something good for your body and mind. Perhaps you would like to give yoga a try, but you don't know where to start. I understand these concerns, so I have developed a simple routine which stretches the whole body, calms the mind and is suitable for yoga beginners.

The below sequence is my go-to routine which I try to do most days. It stretches my whole body, gets my energy flowing, and gives me a positive outlook for the day. I recommend learning this routine first so that it becomes automatic to you. Once you are comfortable with it and can do it without looking at the book, you can learn other routines described in this book. Of course, you can always go to a specific routine for a specific mood, or if you have a special need.

This routine is suitable for all levels, even beginners. Moms experienced with yoga can add more advanced variations. Everyone can find beauty in this simple practice through concentrating on each movement and its alignment with the breath.

This sequence takes around five minutes and can be extended by adding repetitions. When learning the routine, it might take longer so account for that and repeat the routine a couple of times to become familiar with it.

To turn this routine into a ritual, set a positive intention at the beginning. It makes a difference when you dedicate even a small amount of time to a positive goal and do the activity with a positive mindset. You can also do whatever makes this time a bit more special to you. As mentioned previously, a specific time and space is also important. All this creates a meaningful self-care ritual.

Sequence:
1. DEEP BREATHING
2. HEAD ROLLS
3. SHOULDER ROLLS
4. CAT-COW
5. THREAD-THE-NEEDLE POSE
6. DOWNWARD-FACING DOG POSE
7. MOUNTAIN POSE
8. FORWARD BEND POSE
9. PLANK AND LOW PLANK POSE
10. COBRA OR UPWARD-FACING DOG POSE
11. DOWNWARD-FACING DOG POSE
12. CHILD'S POSE

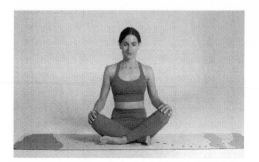

1. DEEP BREATHING
O   This type of breathing calms the mind and
    decreases stress and tension, increas-
    es energy, and lowers blood pressure.
→   Start by sitting in a comfortable seat
    (cross-legged or sitting on your heels) and
    close your eyes. Start by observing how
    your body feels, which parts are touching
    the ground and if - and where - you feel any
    tension. Inhale deeply through your nose
    starting in your belly, through your chest
    and all the way up to your shoulders. Ex-
    hale slowly. Your exhale should take the
    same amount of time as the inhale. This
    slow mindful breathing will help calm you
    down and allow you to be more present.

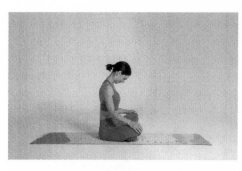
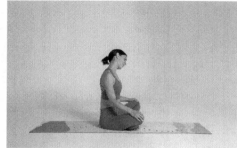

2. HEAD ROLLS
O   Rolling your head stretches the muscles
    around the neck and release any tension.
→   Inhale. Drop your chin towards your chest
    with an exhale. Then roll your head to one
    side while inhaling and do the same on
    the other side. First do the half rolls and
    then the full head rolls. Do it both ways.

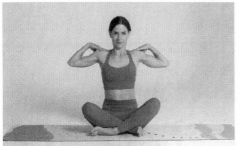
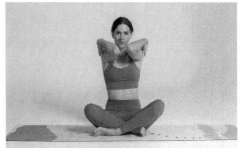
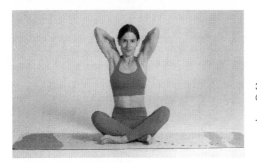

3. ROLLING SHOULDERS
O   This pose stretches the shoulders and acti-
    vates the arms for the upcoming exercise.
→   Start rolling your shoulders. Put your
    hands on your shoulders and draw
    circles with your arms, inhaling and
    exhaling slowly throughout.

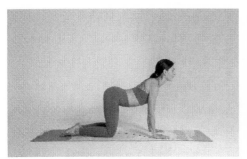
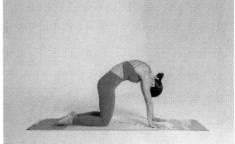

4. CAT-COW POSE
O   Cat-cow stretches the whole neck and
    spine, while having a calming effect.
→   Move so you are on all fours. Hands are
    directly underneath your shoulders and
    knees are under your hips. Your core is
    engaged, and your belly button should be
    slightly pulled in. Your back is straight.

→   Do a simple cat-cow stretch. Inhaling
    through your nose, drop your belly, open
    your chest, looking up and exhale, round-
    ing your spine, chin towards your chest.
→   Continue to wake up your spine and body. Re-
    peat a couple of times. You can add an intuitive
    movement by closing your eyes, moving sideways,
    stretching your spine and back in any way you feel.

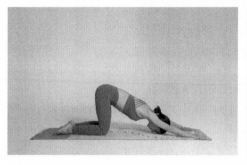
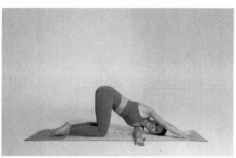

5. THREAD-THE-NEEDLE POSE

O This pose relieves upper back pain, stretches the muscles around your shoulder blades, opens the shoulders and the chest.

→ Extend your arms and place your forehead toward the mat. Keep your back straight and activate your core by bringing your belly in.

→ Bring your left arm under your right. Breathe into your upper back and relax the area between your shoulder blades. Take a few deep breaths, then repeat on the other side. Then go back into all fours position.

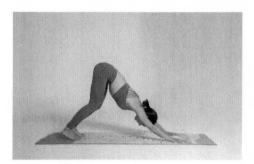

6. DOWNWARD-FACING DOG

O This pose works on strengthening the whole body and stretching the back, legs, and spine.

→ Extend both arms in front of you and spread your fingers. Tuck your toes under and go slowly into Downward-facing Dog by engaging your lower belly on an exhale. Make sure to pull your navel back to your spine. Press through your hands into the mat and push your hips back and up. You should be upside-down in a V shape.

→ Keep your knees bent a little, pedal through your feet to find the length of the spine. Slide your shoulder blades back, and make sure that your neck and jaw are relaxed. Try to bring your heels down towards the mat even if they do not touch the floor. It is not important; the key thing is the intention. Breathe in and out through your nose for 5 breaths.

→ Then step forward in-between your hands and slowly roll vertebra-by-vertebra to Mountain Pose.

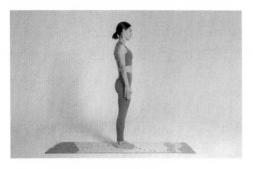

7. MOUNTAIN POSE

O Mountain Pose improves the posture and body alignment.

→ Ground your feet into the mat, making sure to press through all the corners of your feet. Your feet should be together or hip width apart. Tuck your tailbone slightly. Do not round your lower back and pull your belly button in slightly. Lengthen your spine and draw your shoulder blades away from your head.

→ Your arms should be by your side with your fingers wide. Lengthen your neck, and with each inhale try to imagine being tall and straight as if someone is pulling you up using a string.

→ Take a deep breath in and reach both arms up. Exhale and bend forward.

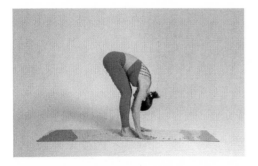

8. FORWARD BEND

O This is a wonderful pose for keeping your spine flexible, relieving tension in the back, while building up strength in the lower body.

→ Your knees are loose and not locked. Your spine is rounded and relaxed. Take deep breaths throughout. If possible, bring your fingertips or palms to your ankles, or to the floor next to your feet. Alternatively, hold your elbows while crossing your forearms.

O While bending forward, straighten your back (you can place your hands on your thighs, under your knees or all the way on the mat), keeping the spine straight with your shoulder blades together. Breathe in and out slowly. Then go back to the forward bend with a rounded spine.

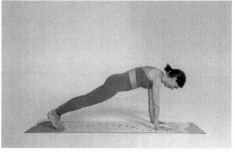

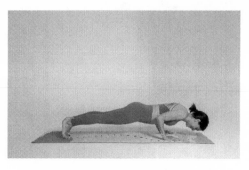

9. PLANK AND LOW PLANK POSE

O These poses are effective for building up strength in your core, arms, and shoulders. They also help with your posture, back pain and boosting your metabolism.

→ Inhale and step back into the Plank Pose. Your body should be in a straight line from head to toe. Imagine drawing a line from your heels to the crown of your head - your hips should not be sticking out. Bring your shoulders over your wrists and spread your fingers wide. Draw your torso forward until it is parallel to the floor. Press your hands into the floor and push your shoulder blades away.

→ Keep your core engaged and tuck your ribs in. Look straight down with no pressure on the back of your neck. Hold for one inhale and then exhale.

→ Keep pushing your heels back and into the floor as if you were pressing against a wall.

→ Relax your jaw muscles and slightly look forward.

→ Low plank - Shift the plank forward and move your shoulders in front of your wrists. Move your feet up until you are on your tippy toes. Bend your elbows straight back as you hug them to the side of your body as you lower into low plank. Pause for one inhale and exhale at the bottom before lying on your stomach.

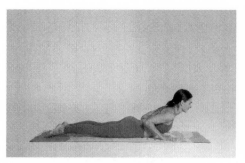

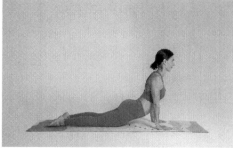

10. COBRA POSE/UPWARD-FACING DOG

O This invigorating backbend helps with strengthening your entire back and shoulders, toning your abdomen, and helping with the flexibility of your spine.

→ Lower your body from Low Plank and lay on your stomach. Your legs should be stretched back with your toes pointing straight back. Your elbows should be bent and close to the body. Put your hands underneath your shoulders.

→ As you inhale, press your hands into the mat and lift your chest up. Press your shoulder blades into your back to open your chest. Move your hands to find the position where the backbend feels comfortable to you. Draw your upper arm bones back and lengthen your neck.

→ Engage the core to protect the lower back in this pose. Keep your thighs firm, arms strong and your elbow bent facing forward. Look straight ahead or tip your head back slightly, but do not compress the back of your neck.

→ Alternatively, in the Upward-facing Dog variation, your arms are straight and keep your shoulders away from your ears.

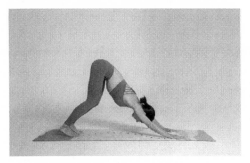

11. DOWNWARD-FACING DOG
O   This pose can also have a calming ef-
     fect and stimulate blood circulation.
→   Inhale and move again into the Down-
     ward-facing Dog, then exhale. See
     Step 6 for full instructions.
→   Take three deep breaths in this pose.

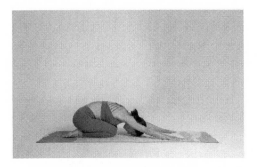

12. CHILD'S POSE
O   This pose lengthens and stretches the
     spine, relaxes your body, and releases
     tension in your back, shoulders, and chest.
→   At the end of the practice, lower your knees
     to the ground and then spread them apart.
     Release your torso in between your thighs
     and rest your forehead on the mat. Relax
     in this position for five breaths. Your hands
     can be extended or next to your torso.
O   If you wish to have a longer practice and
     want to repeat the flow, you can do it again
     from Mountain Pose, Cobra, then Down-
     ward-facing Dog (steps 7-11) three times.

This short routine will activate your whole body and leave you feeling
refreshed with new energy.

Standard Calming Micro-yoga Routine

Moms can feel very exhausted after a day full of balancing all the duties with their family, job, and household.

This quick routine is perfect for the evening before going to bed, especially after a long and stressful day. All the following poses should be done slowly, mindfully and with minimal effort.

Ideally, you should have your eyes closed. Your attention should be on your breathing and on releasing all parts of your body. In case of any discomfort, you may use yoga blocks or other objects for support for any of the exercises. It is useful to let the gravity and exhalation help you with releasing any tension while in any of the poses.

Sequence:
1.   HEAD TO KNEE POSE
2.   KING PIGEON POSE
3.   WIDE-ANGLE SEATED FORWARD BEND POSE
4.   WHOLE BODY SIDE STRETCH
5.   BELLY TWIST

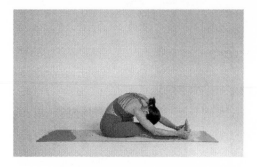

1. HEAD TO KNEE POSE
O   This pose is great for calming the mind, stim-
    ulating digestion, as well as relieving men-
    strual aches. It is also wonderful for stretch-
    ing the back of the body, hips, and groins.
→   Sit with your legs outstretched in front of you.
→   Bend your left leg and place the left
    foot against the left inner thigh.
→   Flex your right foot and raise
    your arms above your head.

→   Turn slightly towards your right leg
    and with an exhale fold forward.
→   Hold your ankle or foot or place
    your hands next to your leg. If
    your extended knee feels un-
    comfortable, bend it slightly.
→   Try keeping your spine long while
    breathing deep. Shoulders are relaxed
    and chest open. After 5 deep breaths
    gently come out of the pose.

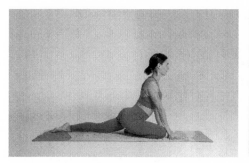
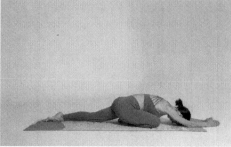

2. KING PIGEON POSE
O   Benefits of this back-bend pose include
    stretching your hip flexors, groin muscles
    and thigh muscles. It is also beneficial
    for opening the shoulders and chest.
→   Start on all fours, then bring your right knee
    forward toward your right wrist. Your knee
    may be just behind your wrist or on the outer
    or the inner edge of it. Your right ankle should
    be in front of your left hip. Notice how you
    feel in this position and what stretch you feel
    in your hips without any tension in your knee.
→   Slide your left leg back, pointing your toes,
    and point your heel up towards the ceiling.
→   Keep your hips square by drawing your
    legs in towards each other. You can use
    some support under your right buttock
    if needed, to keep your hips level.
→   Breathe in and come onto your finger-
    tips; lengthen your spine, draw your
    belly button in and open your chest.

→   Breathe out, lower your upper body
    towards the floor. You can rest on your
    forearms, or with your forehead on the mat
    with extended arms. If your forehead does
    not reach the mat, you can make fists with
    your hands and stack them on each other
    and rest your forehead on your hands.
→   Stay for 5 breaths. As you exhale, release
    any tension you might feel in your right hip.
→   Push back through your hands, lift
    your hips, and move your leg back
    to come back to the starting posi-
    tion. Repeat on the other side.
→   This can still be quite an intense pose,
    especially for your outer hip. Try keep-
    ing your right foot close to your left
    hip to start with. The more your shin is
    parallel with the front of the mat, the
    more intense the hip opener will be.
→   Always listen to your body and how it
    feels, without pushing through the pain.

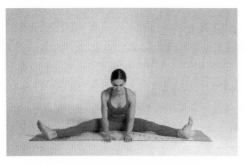

spread your legs wide apart until you feel a good stretch in your legs. Keep your spine straight and your feet flexed.

→ Lengthen up through your spine – imagine as if someone is holding your spine on a string. Bend from the hips and place your hands on the mat between your legs. Then slowly exhale and walk your hands forward.

→ As you go lower into the forward bend, still maintain a long spine. If your back arches, do not go down any further. Hold this pose for 5 breaths.

→ To come out of the pose, come up with a straight back.

→ Your current range of motion might not allow you to bring your torso too much forward to the mat. In that case, you can bend your knees a little. You can also take a rolled blanket and lay it in front of you. Exhale into the forward bend and lay your torso down on this support. Be kind to yourself and accept your current flexibility.

3. WIDE-ANGLE SEATED FORWARD BEND
O This calming pose is great for opening your entire back and increasing the range of motion in your hips, lower back, and hamstrings.
→ If you have a lower-back injury, sit up high on a folded blanket, and keep your torso relatively upright.
→ Start seated with your legs straight. Then

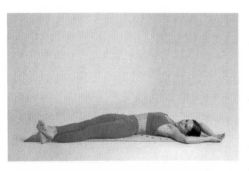

back issues, you might not want to go too deep into this pose.

→ Lie on your back with your legs straight on the floor. Reach your arms overhead and clasp your hands. Then move your feet and upper body to the right. Arch your back like a ripe banana.

→ Do not twist or roll your hips off the mat. Find your comfortable stretch. Then try moving your feet further to the right as well as your whole upper body.

→ Cross your ankles to get a deeper stretch. Inhale and exhale 5 times.

→ To come out of the pose, bring your legs to the centre and your arms down. After, hug your knees towards your chest and make gentle circles for a few breaths.

4. WHOLE BODY SIDE STRETCH
O This is a great side bend that stretches your back muscles and the whole side of your body. If you have lower

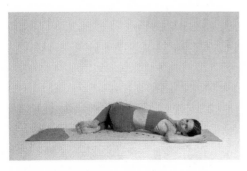

→ Lie on your back and extend your arms to the sides with palms facing down. Bend both knees to your chest.

→ With an exhale, drop both knees over to the right. You might feel a slight twisting of your spine. Slide your knees as close to your right arm as possible and turn your head to the left.

→ Keep your shoulders flat on the floor, close your eyes and relax into the posture. Let gravity pull your knees down. Use the right hand on the left knee to pull your knees down. You can place a blanket under your knees in case of any tension. Stay in this position for 5 breaths.

→ To release, inhale and roll the hips back to the floor. Repeat on the other side.

5. BELLY TWIST
O This is a great spinal and belly twist that stretches the back muscles, lengthens the spine, and hydrates the spinal disks.

After this short winding-down routine, you might feel nicely relaxed with a restored calm and feel ready for the rest of the day. Again, you can turn this exercise into a small ritual by making the place and time special for you. For instance, by engaging your senses through smell, sound, and sight. Think about using a scented candle, playing gentle instrumental music, or reading a positive quote before your practice.

In the next chapter, I will introduce a few energizing Micro-yoga routines that are suitable for times when we need a dynamic practice.

Energizing Micro-yoga Routines

We all have days when we feel we can conquer the world and we feel particularly strong and bold. On those days, we might want to try a more powerful exercise to strengthen our bodies. On such days, it is suitable to choose an energizing micro-routine based on more dynamic yoga styles.

In this chapter, I will introduce a few routines that have an energizing potential and can still be done within circa five minutes. In this short amount of time, these powerful energizing sequences can activate our bodies, lift our spirit, and re-energize our entire body.

Tremendous benefits that these energizing micro-routines can bring include:

→ Boosting energy.
→ Waking up the body and mind.
→ Strengthening the muscles.
→ Building up stamina.

Optimal Timing:

→ Before everyone wakes up and before you have your morning shower.
→ During your child's naptime.
→ During a mid-afternoon energy slump to boost energy.
→ After coming from work to increase the energy levels for the evening.
→ Before dinner to increase metabolism.
→ Anytime that works best for your rhythm in your family and when you can dedicate at least five minutes for your practice.

Energizing Core Micro-yoga Workout

Whenever I want to work on my core strength, get an energetic boost and give my muscles a more powerful workout, I do this five-minute core routine. It might involve a bit of sweat, but it is worth it for the physical strength and stamina.

Here are a few yoga asanas that will energize the whole body and make the core muscles work in just a few minutes.

Sequence:
1. BALANCING TABLE POSE.
2. KNEES OFF THE FLOOR.
3. PLANK POSE.
4. BENDING KNEES IN PLANK.
5. SIDE PLANK POSE.
6. CHILD'S POSE.
7. ONE-LEGGED DOWNWARD-FACING DOG WITH BENDING KNEES.
8. CHILD'S POSE.

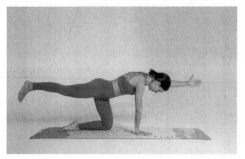

1. BALANCING TABLE POSE
O   This pose engages your core and strength-
    ens your balance and concentration.
→   Start on all fours. Put your hands direct-
    ly beneath your shoulders. Make sure
    your knees line up with your hips. Your
    back is straight, and your core is en-
    gaged, belly button pulling inward.
→   Inhale and extend your left arm and right leg.
    Exhale and hold. Hold for 5 breaths while
    breathing deeply. Then switch legs and arms.

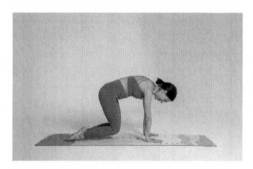

2. KNEES OFF THE FLOOR
O   This exercise builds up abdominal
    and arm and shoulder muscles.
→   Still on all fours, inhale and bring your
    knees up a few centimetres off the floor.
    Exhale. Then hold for five breaths. En-
    gage the core, keeping your back
    straight throughout the exercise.

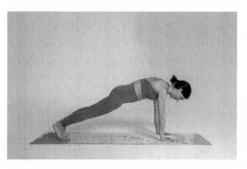

3. PLANK POSE
O   This pose is effective for building up
    strength in your core, arms, and shoulders.
→   Hold for 5 breaths.
→   For full instructions see Stand-
    ard Energizing Routine.

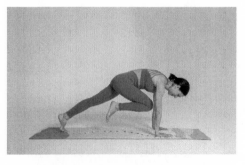

4. BENDING KNEES IN PLANK
O   This is a powerful exercise for build-
    ing your core strength.
→   Inhale. With an exhale, bend your right knee
    and bring it towards your chest. Exhale. Switch
    legs, bringing your left knee towards your
    chest. Repeat six times on each side. If six
    times is too much, repeat twice on each side.
→   You can also do it while being on your
    forearms. Still in Plank or Forearm Plank,
    inhale and bend your right knee. With an
    exhalation, bring it towards the opposite
    elbow. Switch sides. Repeat six times.

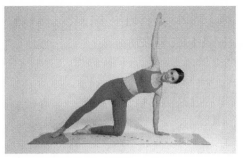

5. SIDE PLANK
O   This is a brilliant full-body exercise. It strengthens the oblique ab muscles, arms, wrists, and
legs. It builds balance, focus and coordination.
→   Open to the right side, balancing on your left
hand and right outer foot. Keep left leg bent
for better support. Alternatively, stack your
ankles on top of each other or put your feet
next to each other on the mat. Point your right
arm at the ceiling. Stack your hand over your
ear. Do not let it fall behind. Your tailbone
should be directed towards your heels.
→   Hold for 5 breaths and then switch sides.

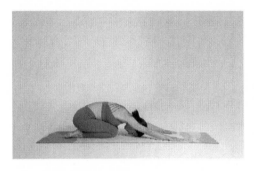

6. CHILD'S POSE
O   This pose lengthens and stretches the
spine, relaxes your body, and releases
tension in your back, shoulders, and chest.
→   Take a break for a couple of deep
breaths. For full instructions, see
Standard Energizing Routine.

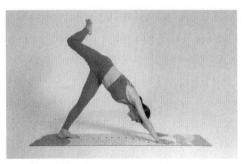

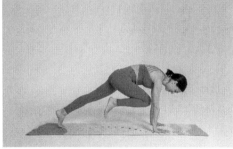

7. ONE-LEGGED DOWNWARD-FACING
DOG WITH BENDING KNEES TOWARD
THE ELBOWS
→   Go into Downward-facing Dog (see Stand-
ard Energizing Routine for a reminder).

Breathe in and extend your right leg. Then
bend your right knee. Exhale and bring
your right knee towards your right elbow.
Repeat six times and then switch legs.

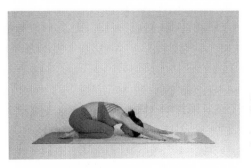

8. CHILD'S POSE
O   This is a great relaxation pose suita-
ble for the end of the sequence.
→   See step 6 above.
→   Move your knees down to the floor
and rest in this pose for 10 breaths.

After this dynamic practice, you might be breathing quickly, but your energy should be flowing more freely in your body, and you might feel a rush of endorphins in your brain. If the repetitions feel too challenging at the beginning, start with lower repetitions but try all the exercises. If one of the exercises feel particularly tough, you can skip it, do the rest, and give it a try next time.

As always, the most important part is to show up, honour your body, notice what sensations you feel during the routine and try as much as you can each day.

Energizing Micro-yoga Flow

This is a swift yoga flow that increases the energy flowing in your body and gets your body nicely stretched and revitalized. It is called a flow because there is a beautiful alliance between movement and breath as you move through the poses in this sequence. Repeat the sequence twice, first starting with the right side in the high lunge and then on the left side.

Sequence:
1. CHAIR POSE
2. HIGH LUNGE POSE
3. WARRIOR 2 POSE
4. REVERSE WARRIOR POSE
5. EXTENDED SIDE ANGLE POSE
6. TRIANGLE POSE
7. WARRIOR 1 POSE WITH T-ARMS
8. PLANK POSE
9. UPWARD-FACING DOG POSE
10. DOWNWARD-FACING DOG POSE
11. FORWARD BEND POSE
12. MOUNTAIN POSE

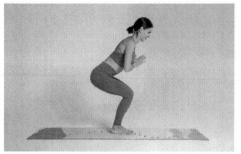
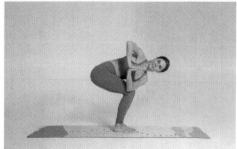

1. CHAIR POSE

O This pose delivers various benefits; from strengthening your thighs and ankles, while toning your shoulders, butt, hips, and back. It also stretches the shoulders and opens the chest, increasing your breathing capacity and improving your posture.

→ Start in Chair Pose. Before going into the squat, find the centre of your balance in each foot. Then exhale and bend your knees and send your glutes down, as if you are sitting on an imaginary chair. Press your legs gently toward each other and press your hips toward your midline.

When you can no longer maintain the stable centre in your feet, stop bending your knees.

→ Place your palms together in front of your chest. Draw your lower ribs in and do not overarch your lower back. Open your chest and rotate your shoulders away from your ears. Take a deep breath in and out a couple times. Release the pose and move your feet so you do not get cramps.

→ Chair To the Side: With palms together in front of your chest, rotate to the right. Your left elbow is next to your right knee, and your knees are in the centre together and are not leaning to the side. Take a few deep breaths and then rotate to the left.

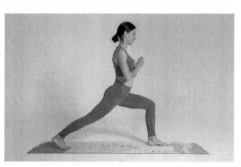

2. HIGH LUNGE POSE

O This pose stretches your ankles, calves, hamstrings, opens your hips, and builds up strength in your legs as well as shoulders and arms.

→ Exhale and step your right foot back. Your heel is off the floor and your left leg is strong. Keep your left knee over your heel. Do not overarch your lower back.

→ Take a few deep breaths and then align your feet into Warrior 2.

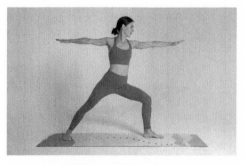

3. WARRIOR 2

O Warrior 2 enhances strength, stability, and concentration. It is also a great stretch for the legs, groin, and chest. It strengthens your thigh and glute muscles.

→ Align your heels. Your right foot should be at 90 degrees, with your toes pointing to the top of the mat. Your back foot should be at a 45-degree angle.

→ Raise your arms out to your side at shoulder height, parallel to the floor. Your arms should be aligned directly over your legs with your palms facing down.

→ Your front knee should be bent and directly over the ankle of your front foot. Sink your hips low, bringing your front thigh parallel to the floor, if possible. Your knee should not move past your ankle.

→ Keep your back leg straight, lift your chest and drop your shoulders. Keep your arms active and your gaze focused on your middle finger.

→ Take 5 deep breaths and release the pose. Lower your arms and straighten your front leg. Continue to the next pose.

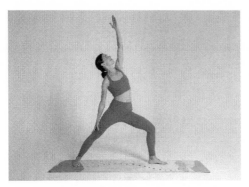

4. REVERSE WARRIOR
O   This is a wonderful stretch for your legs, groins, hips, sides of your torso and waist. It increases blood flow throughout your body, reducing tiredness and calming the mind.
→   From Warrior 2 on your next exhale, drop your back hand to the back of your right thigh. On an inhale, lift your left arm up, reaching the fingers towards the ceiling. Keeping your front knee bent and sink low as you slide your left hand down your left leg. Your gaze is on your left fingertips. You should feel a gentle backbend in this pose. Relax your shoulders, open your chest, and hold this pose for 5 deep breaths.

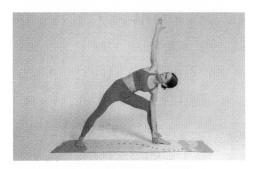

5. EXTENDED SIDE ANGLE POSE
O   This pose is wonderful for stretching the whole side of your body as well as your inner thighs and groin. It relieves lower back pain and menstrual pain. Also, it improves stamina and strengthens your leg muscles.
→   From the Reverse Warrior Pose, go into an extended side angle by extending your left arm and then placing your left hand outside of your left foot. Or you can place it on your left knee, depending on your flexibility. Extend your right arm up to the sky. With an inhale, flip your palm to face the floor and reach your right arm overhead. Draw your shoulders away from your ears, stretch through your side body and open your chest. Your gaze should be toward your right arm.
→   Take 5 deep breaths and then release the pose by returning into Warrior 2.

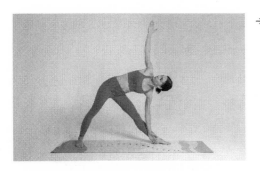

6. TRIANGLE POSE
O   This is an energizing pose for strengthening your legs and back, stretching your hamstrings, calves, spine, and shoulders. It also opens your chest and hips.
→   From the Warrior 2 pose, straighten your left leg while keeping a micro-bend. Then inhale as you reach to the left, extending your body over your left leg. As you do this, shift your hips towards the back of the mat. Exhale as you bring your left arm down, placing your hand either on your left leg, the mat, or a block. Rotate your chest towards the ceiling and look up if your neck is comfortable. If not, look straight ahead. Your neck should be in line with your spine. Reach your left arm straight up to the ceiling, in line with your shoulder, and face your palms forward.
→   Stay in this position for 5 deep breaths.
→   To come out, inhale and reach your left arm up to the ceiling as you come back into Warrior 2. Then move into Warrior 1.

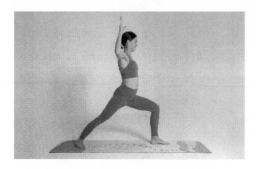

7.	WARRIOR 1 WITH T-ARMS
O	This energizing pose delivers multiple benefits from strengthening your legs, arms, and shoulder muscles to opening your chest and lungs. This encourages good breathing and improves stability and concentration.
→	From Warrior 2, align your hips with the front edge of the mat so that they are squared. Your upper body should be facing the front edge of the mat and your shoulders should be far away from your ears. Your left knee should be bent, parallel to the floor, with your back foot grounded and engaged.
→	Tuck your belly in, lengthen your spine and put your arms into a T, opening your chest. Breathe deeply in and out for 5 breaths. Then lower your arms, inhale, and step into Plank Pose.

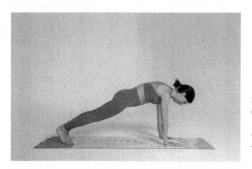

8.	PLANK POSE
O	This pose is great for building up strength in your core, arms, and shoulders.
→	One deep breath in and out.
→	For full instructions, see Stand-ard Energizing Routine.

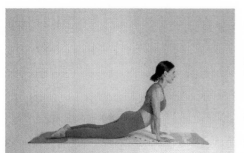

9.	UPWARD-FACING DOG
O	This invigorating backbend helps with strengthening your entire back and shoulders, toning your abdomen, and helping with the flexibility of your spine.
→	Inhale and move into Down-ward-Facing dog, exhale.
→	For full instructions, see Stand-ard Energizing Routine.

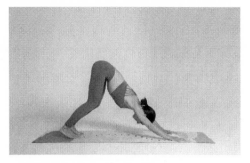

10. DOWNWARD-FACING DOG
O   This pose works on strengthen-
    ing the whole body and stretch-
    ing the back, legs, and spine.
→   Couple inhales and exhales in this pose.
→   For full instructions, see Stand-
    ard Energizing Routine.

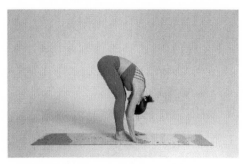

11. FORWARD BEND
O   This pose stretches the hamstrings, knees,
    and hips. It activates your abdominal muscles
    and stretches and strengthens your spine.
→   On an inhale, lift and lengthen the torso.
    On an exhale, release more into the fold.
→   For full instructions, see Standard En-
    ergizing Routine. Breathe in and out.

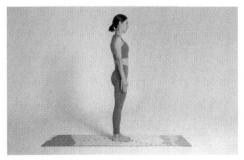

12. MOUNTAIN POSE
O   This pose improves the pos-
    ture and body alignment.
→   Roll slowly vertebra-by-verte-
    bra to the Mountain Pose.
→   Place your hands by your side or
    palms in front of your chest and
    breathe in and out deeply.

You can repeat the whole sequence on the other side with the left leg extended in the High Lunge Pose. Depending on how fast you go through the poses, the sequence can be quite energizing and strengthening the whole body, leaving you feeling strong, stretched and in control.

Energizing Micro-yoga Inversion Practice

Inversions are yoga poses where the head is below the heart. There are many benefits to trying to incorporate these inversions into your life. These include eliminating toxins, boosting energy and improving immunity. In addition to this, inversions increase the oxygen flow into the brain, improve circulation and stimulate your nervous system. They also calm the mind, strengthen the back and core abdominal muscles, improve overall posture and balance.

When to utilize these inversions:
1. In the morning to start your day with a high energy boost.
2. During a mid-afternoon energy slump to boost energy.
3. When you want to get a new perspective on something.
4. When you want to stimulate your brain and decrease fatigue.
5. After coming home from work to increase energy levels for the evening.

Of course, as with any yoga practice, it is not just about turning yourself upside down but about doing it mindfully while concentrating on your breath. Only this way, the practice brings its benefits.

There are a few contraindications with inversions, so we need to be mindful about our health conditions before starting this practice. The best advice is to double check your condition with your doctor before practising inversions and work with a doctor and a yoga teacher to adapt positions. For instance, people with high blood pressure, heart conditions or asthma, and some back conditions, should avoid any inverted positions.

For moms, it is always debated about whether we should practice inversions when we have a period. I would suggest doing a little research for yourself. Again, we should listen to our bodies and see what feels good for us. For me, usually simple inverted postures are ok, but I do not enjoy an advanced inversion as much.

There are two types of yoga inversions with heating or cooling effect. Those with a heating effect on the body are usually more advanced and energizing (think of a Headstand, Handstand, etc.) and the cooling ones with a calming effect are usually more accessible for beginners.

In this section, we will explore some simple energizing inversions that are still suitable for those who are starting with yoga and yet still have the benefits of the more advanced inversions.

ENERGIZING MICRO-YOGA INVERSION SEQUENCE

When I feel sluggish in the afternoon, I sometimes try an inversion to bring my head below the heart. Typical inversions I do quite often are Headstands and Shoulder Stands, but there are more yoga asanas accessible for those beginning with their yoga journey. I will explore these in the following Micro-yoga practice.

Sequence:
1. DOWNWARD-FACING DOG
2. DOWNWARD-FACING DOG WITH A TWIST
3. TRIPOD HEADSTAND PREPARATION
4. CHILD'S POSE

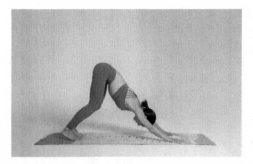

1. DOWNWARD-FACING DOG
O   Downward Dog is a simple inversion pose for beginners as the head is below the heart and you will get all the benefits of the inversion. It is a beneficial pose as it stretches the hamstrings and calf muscles in the back of your legs, and it builds shoulder strength.
→   Breathe in and out 5 times or for about one minute.
→   For full instructions, see Standard Energizing routine.

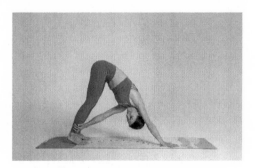

2. DOWNWARD -FACING DOG WITH A TWIST
O   This pose has the same benefits as the regular Down dog with added rotation that increases the spine mobility.
→   Keep your right hand grounded into the mat and touch your right ankle or calf with your left hand. Keep gazing to your right. You should feel a stretch on the left side of your body. Keep your knees soft and press heels to the mat to deepen the stretch.
→   With every exhale, deepen a bit more into the twist. Take 5 deep breaths. Inhale and with the next exhale, come back to Downward-facing dog. Repeat on the other side.

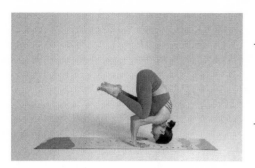

3. TRIPOD HEAD STAND PREPARATION
O   This preparation pose will energize
    your mind while strengthening your
    core, back, neck, shoulders as well as
    easing pressure on your lower back.
→   There is no experience needed for this
    Headstand preparation pose. Head-
    stands might make you feel uncom-
    fortable, but after trying this and
    succeeding, you will feel like you do
    not have to be afraid of them at all.
→   To begin with, try doing this Headstand
    facing the wall for the added safe-
    ty. Once you feel stronger, try to do
    it a bit further from the wall, perhaps
    with someone who can support you.
→   Start in the Tabletop position. Make
    sure that your shoulders are di-

rectly above your wrists, and your
hips are right above your knees.
→   Bend your elbows at a 90-degree angle
    and place the top of your head on the
    floor in front of your hands. You should
    be able to see your fingertips. Your hands
    and head will form a tripod. Remem-
    ber, a strong foundation for this pose is
    more important than the final goal.
→   Curl your toes and lift your knees off the
    floor. Start walking your feet in towards
    your hands so that your hips are lifted
    high into the air. Notice how you feel. If
    your hamstrings hurt, come back to this
    pose after you have stretched. If your
    neck feels tight, try lengthening your
    neck while you draw your shoulders away
    from your ears. If the top of your head
    hurts, adjust your balance point a bit. Find
    the right spot for your own body.
→   Make sure that your elbows continue to point
    in the same direction that you are facing.
→   Slowly try lifting one knee and placing it
    onto one of the triceps. It is ok to stay here
    if you do not wish to continue. If you still
    feel comfortable and stable, slowly lift your
    other foot from the floor and place the knee
    on the back of your other tricep. Remem-
    ber to keep your neck long and breathe
    deeply. You have reached the Headstand
    preparation pose. Take 5 deep breaths,
    then come out slowly out of the pose.

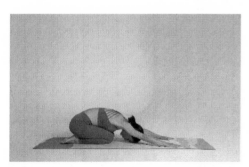

4. CHILD'S POSE
O   This is a wonderful relaxation pose
    for the end of any sequence.
→   Complete this sequence with
    a relaxing Child's pose.
→   For full instructions, see Standard Energizing
    Routine. Take 5 deep breaths in and out.
→   After this pose, you can slowly move your
    body into the upright position. Stand tall
    and straight while you take a few deep
    breaths with hands in front of your heart.

Thank yourself for taking the time to care for your body and mind
today. Breathe in and out deeply and notice how different you
might feel after this short inversion practice.

Calming Micro-yoga Practices

There are many days when we feel exhausted and stressed out due to balancing all the responsibilities we have. On those days, we do not have the mood to push ourselves for a dynamic exercise and our bodies might crave something gentler and slower. Calming yoga practices provide a wonderful solution for such times when we do not have much energy left. This is also an important part of the yoga journey as well as our own self-care; to be able to incorporate restorative practices into our days. Even a short time alone and undisturbed in a gentle yoga pose can do wonders. It re-balances our body and mind and leaves us feeling calmer.

I certainly use these calming Micro-yoga practices on those days when it is all a bit too much for me and I have little energy left. Because I still want to do something good for my body and mind, this is when I turn to a nice relaxation exercise, or a quick breathing exercise. Even just five minutes of a slower-paced self-care routine leaves me feeling relaxed and allows me to be able to care for others.

There are numerous benefits of calming yoga routines:
→ Relaxing the body.
→ Lowering blood pressure and heart rate.
→ Calming your mind.
→ Easing anxiety and reducing stress.

When to do it:
→ When feeling anxious, stressed out, or overwhelmed by childcare and other duties.
→ When we need to find our centre and focus.
→ A way to relax after an exhausting day.
→ When we want to focus on the present moment.

There are many different yoga practices that have a calming effect on our bodies and mind. These include restorative yoga, balancing and inversion asanas, relaxation, and breathing techniques.

Next, I will introduce a Micro-yoga sequence from each of these calming practices, created for all busy moms, at all levels of fitness and range of motion.

Calming Balance Micro-yoga Routine

Balance poses are yoga positions where we need to engage our core and focus on concentration to be able to stay in balance. Thus, their main physical benefits are strengthening the core and improving the entire posture. The mental benefits include improving concentration and having a calming effect on our mood.

When performing balance asanas, it is recommended to look at one stable point in front of your eyes to help you maintain stability. Also, deep breathing helps as it naturally calms down the nervous system. This is because breathing slowly engages the parasympathetic nervous system. This type of breathing also helps your stability in the poses.

The balancing poses also benefit our mental state and influence our mind. A study has shown that inner focus and balance cause changes in brainwaves, resulting in a more meditative state of mind (Liou, 2010).

When I am short of time and want to calm myself down, I do this super quick Micro-yoga routine. I also do it when I have a long to-do list, or I need to have an important conversation. This sequence is great for focused mindset that is needed for all moms. It takes around five minutes, and it is suitable for all fitness levels.

If you do not feel very stable today, feel free to try this sequence by standing next to a wall or a piece of furniture. If you want to try a challenge, you can try the whole sequence of three poses one after another without touching your foot to the ground. First try with one leg and then repeat with the other one.

Sequence:
1. HEAD-TO-KNEE PREPARATION POSE
2. STANDING TWIST BALANCE POSE
3. DANCER'S POSE
4. TREE POSE

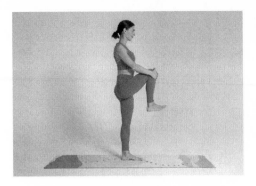

1. HEAD-TO-KNEE PREPARATION POSE
O This pose is wonderful for calming your brain and stretching your spine, shoulders, hamstrings, and groin. It also improves digestion and relieves anxiety, tiredness, and headaches, as well as menstrual discomfort.
→ Notice your feet on the mat - imagine they are the roots of a stable tree.
→ Stand tall with your spine straight and gaze forward. Make sure your feet are together, and slightly engage your core by pulling your belly button towards your spine. Your shoulders should be far apart and pulled away from the ears.
→ Inhale slowly. Bend your right leg and pull your knee towards your chest and exhale. Either stay still or try rotating your right ankle. From a standing position, your weight should be balanced on one leg while your other leg is bent at the knee and pulled in towards the torso. Your palms can be on the knee, on your shin, or under the sole of the foot with your fingers interlaced under your foot. Breathe in and out 5 times and then release the pose. Repeat with the other leg.

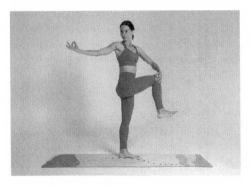

2. STANDING TWIST BALANCE
O This is a wonderful pose for strengthening the flexibility of the spine and waist. It develops focus and awareness of the core. It builds up arm and leg muscles.
→ In the Head-to-Knee Preparation Pose, place your left palm on your right knee and rotate from your navel and ribcage as you extend your right arm behind you.
→ Your left hand should grasp your right knee. Open your chest and breathe deeply. Gaze behind you.
→ Try to distribute your weight evenly across the planted foot to help with balance. Adding a twist and a gaze behind you forces you to quiet your mind and focus, and it engages the core. Take 5 deep breaths and try not to hold your breath. Then release and repeat on the other side.

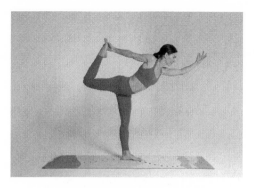

3.　DANCER'S POSE

O　This is a brilliant balance pose that builds the strength in your core and legs. It also stretches your shoulders and hip flexors.

→　Stand tall with both feet on the mat. Then inhale and put your right leg behind you. Catch your right foot in your right palm firmly - your hand can either be on the inside or outside of your foot. Your right and left knee should be tucked together. Exhale slowly.

→　Inhale and extend your left arm above your head. With a slow exhalation, start moving slowly down with your torso, parallel to the mat and start to extend your right leg behind you. Breathe slowly and mindfully to maintain your stability. Inhale in and exhale out 5 times.

→　Slowly with control, release the pose and return to the centre. Your left arm should move downwards and mindfully return your right leg to the floor.

→　Repeat on the other side.

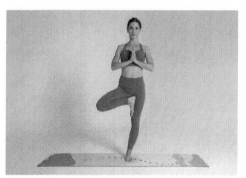

4.　TREE POSE

O　Tree Pose is a fantastic balance exercise for building up strength in your legs and core. It increases flexibility in your hips and stretches your inner thighs and groin muscles. It is a wonderful pose for after a long day sitting and helps with relieving anxious thoughts by calming your mind.

→　As a beginner, you can use a wall to help keep your balance. You can then try it without the wall later.

→　Stand tall with a straight spine and ground your feet into the mat underneath you. Make sure your weight is distributed equally on all sides of each foot.

→　Shift your weight onto your left foot, imagining as if it is a root of a tree. Lift your right foot off the mat. Keep your left leg straight without locking your knee.

→　Bend your right knee and bring the sole of your right foot high onto your inner left thigh (or your left calf or ankle, depending on where you feel the most stable). Do what feels right to your body. Do not place the foot on the side of the knee as this puts your joint in a vulnerable position.

→　Hips should stay square toward the front, so your right hip does not stick out.

→　To help with your balance, focus your gaze on something that does not move. When you are in the Tree Pose, you can put your hands together in front of your chest.

→　Inhale and exhale deeply 5 times, then release the pose and stand tall with your feet together. Pedal the feet to avoid cramps. Then repeat on the other side.

At the end of the sequence, stand tall in the Mountain Pose with your eyes closed and take a few deep breaths. Notice how this sequence has made you feel and whether you feel more focused and calmer.

Calming Micro-yoga Inversion Practice

All the exercises in this sequence are inversions suitable for beginners who are not familiar with being upside down in yoga. This sequence has a calming effect and still brings the benefits of inversions. It is possible to do all these poses in around five minutes. For a more restorative-style practice, choose one of these Asanas and spend the whole five (or more) minutes in one pose.

Sequence:
1.   STANDING FORWARD FOLD – RAG DOLL POSE
2.   PUPPY POSE
3.   SUPPORTED SHOULDER STAND
4.   LEGS UP THE WALL POSE

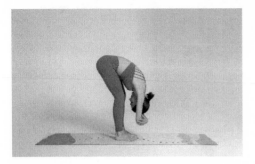

1. STANDING FORWARD FOLD – RAG DOLL POSE

O   This is a great inverted pose for stretching the ankles, calves, hamstrings, and lower back. It also releases tension in your neck and shoulders and can help to ease lower back and neck pain. This pose can also alleviate stress and tension, so it works well for calming purposes.

→   Start in Mountain Pose: Stand up straight and then bend forward, moving into the Standing Forward Bend. Your feet should be hip width apart. If you like, take a generous bend in your knees so that your chest and thighs touch. Feel your weigh in the balls of your feet to send the sit bones up.

→   Hold your opposite elbows. You can start moving slowly side-to-side, while breathing deeply. Take 5 deep breaths. To release the pose, unclasp the elbows and on an inhale, slowly move vertebra-by-vertebra back to the start.

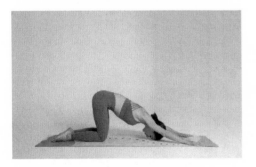

2. PUPPY POSE

O   This is a brilliant and calming near-inversion pose. This pose stretches the upper back, spine, and shoulders. It helps to open the chest and release the tension in the shoulders and neck.

→   Come into Tabletop on all fours. Your hips are stacked directly over your knees, and your shoulders over your wrists. Rest the tops of your feet on the mat with your toes pointing straight back. Your feet are parallel and hip-width apart.

→   On an exhalation, begin to walk your hands out in front of you. Allow your chest to release toward the floor and slowly place your forehead onto the mat.

→   Spread your fingers and press firmly into your thumb and index fingers. Broaden your shoulders by rolling your upper arm bones away from your ears. Your arms are active, and your elbows are lifted slightly off the mat.

→   Inhale and reach your hips up and back; while still letting your chest melt down toward the floor. Gently hug your front ribs in to support your spine and prevent collapsing into your lower back.

→   Take 5 deep breaths.

→   Release the pose by walking your hands back to Tabletop position.

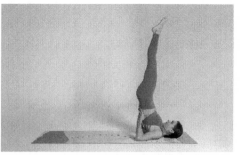

3. SUPPORTED SHOULDER STAND

O Benefits of this pose are tremendous: from stretching the shoulders and neck, reducing the fluid retention in your legs, reducing fatigue, to improving your sleep and calming the nervous system.

→ Lie on your back with your knees bent and your arms alongside your body.

→ On an exhalation, push your lower back into the mat. On an inhale, lift your legs up while you press your arms and palms into the mat.

→ Sweep your legs over your head. Use that momentum to curl your hips up and off the mat. Roll onto your back, bringing your centre of gravity towards your upper back and shoulders.

→ Bend your elbows and place your palms on your back for support. Stretch your legs up towards the ceiling. Draw your elbows in towards each other. Walk your hands up your back, towards your upper back to help lift your spine off the floor. Open your chest and draw your shoulder blades in. Try to keep most of the weight in your upper back and arms.

→ Relax your face and jaw, gaze at your chest and breathe into your belly.

→ To release the pose, lower your legs towards the floor to about a 45-degree angle. Then roll your spine slowly and carefully back onto the floor (with your knees bent if you prefer), eventually placing your feet on the floor.

O The key thing is to take care of your neck. Do not move your neck when you are in the Shoulder Stand. You can also use the wall as a support for your feet. It is also possible to bring your legs to a 45-degree angle instead of extending them up to the ceiling. The position of your elbows is also important. Roll your upper arms outwards to prevent your elbows from splaying out to the sides.

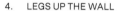

4. LEGS UP THE WALL

O This is another wonderful inversion with a relaxation effect. It is a pose where you can let go of all your stress and anxiety. It can also ease headaches, increase energy, relieve swollen legs, cramps, and lower back pain.

→ Sit with your right side against the wall with your bent knees and your feet drawn in toward your hips.

→ Swing your legs up against the wall as you turn to lie flat on your back.

→ Place your hips against the wall or slightly away. Alternatively, you can keep legs up even if you are not near the wall.

→ Place your arms in any comfortable position.

→ Breathe fully and peacefully taking at least 5 deep inhales and exhales.

→ To come out of the pose, gently push yourself away from the wall.

→ Draw your knees to your chest and roll onto your right side.

→ Take a few deep breaths, then move slowly into a relaxation pose - lying down with legs extended.

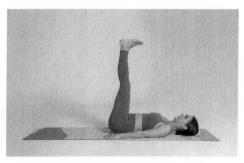

At the end of this practice, stay on the floor with your eyes closed and notice how you feel calmer and more relaxed.

Restorative Micro-yoga

Restorative yoga originally comes from Iyengar yoga, which was developed by yoga master B.K.S. Iyengar. He founded a yoga practice based on the hatha yoga, with more focus on the alignment of yoga poses; using supporting props in asanas that encourage tension and stress release (Norberg, 2016).

Restorative yoga is a technique to help achieve deeper relaxation and greater peace. It elicits the relaxation response, thus re-creating a new balance in our nervous system. We achieve the relaxation response by focusing on the release of the tension in our muscles in longer- held poses.

In this type of yoga practice, we can use different props such as blankets, blocks, bolsters, etc (Yoga Medicine, 2019). A restorative yoga sequence is usually made up of only five or six poses, that are held for five minutes or more. They can help us relax completely (Outside Interactive Inc., 2021).

There are many benefits of the restorative yoga practice. This slow practice can have healing effects on our body and mind. The emphasis is not on stretching, but on releasing the tension and the gentle stimulation of organs. It also teaches us the skills to self-soothe and it enhances the healing capacity of our body (Norberg, 2016).

Restorative yoga can improve our capability to access rest with more ease. Thus, it can reconnect our parasympathetic nervous system. It can also reduce the production of stress hormones, improve sleep, reduce muscle tension, and improve our immune system and have many other benefits (Yoga Medicine, 2019).

Every mom can benefit from the quick restorative yoga routine below. You can always stay longer in the poses or modify them. This is typically advised for this type of practice. In case you only have a few minutes, you can still feel the benefits, especially if you find the time regularly and consistently for this calming practice.

I enjoy this sequence after a long busy day when I know that I do not have much energy left for a more intense routine. On the other hand, it is also great for active relaxation in the middle of the day when I have a few minutes for myself when my kids are asleep.

Sequence:
1. KNEES-TO-CHEST POSE
2. SPINAL TWIST
3. HALF-BRIDGE POSE
4. CORPSE POSE

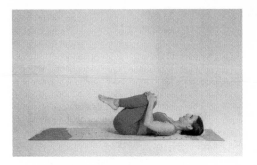

1. KNEES TO CHEST POSE
O This pose releases toxins from the body, releases tension and stimulates internal organs.
→ Start on the ground. Bring your knees to your chest and hold for 30 seconds, with your knees and feet together.
→ Your head should be on the ground. Press your spine into the mat from the base of the skull to the tailbone. This creates stability and allows for increased pressure to be applied to your legs. With your knees pulled to your chest, you can wrap your hands around the tops of the calves and clasp your hands.
→ Breathe in and out deeply 10 times (about 1 minute).

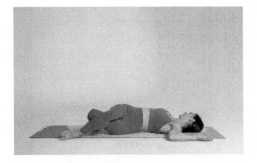

2. SPINAL TWIST
O Spinal Twist has physiological benefits, it stimulates circulation, cleanses organs by releasing toxins, and improves your spine's range of motion.
→ Your arms are stretched out to the sides at shoulder height. Pull your knees up towards your chest. Exhale and drop both knees to one side, keeping your knees pulled up towards your arm. Shoulder blades and shoulders should still be touching the mat.
→ Stay there for 5 breaths. Breathe fully and deeply.
→ On your next exhalation, lift your legs back up towards your chest, flattening your lower back onto the floor. Drop your knees to the other side and breathe deeply for 5 breaths. Then return to the centre.

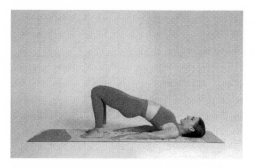

3. HALF-BRIDGE POSE
O   Half-Bridge strengthens abdominal and lumbar muscles, tones your glutes, and legs, and releases lower back tension and pain.
→   Stay lying on your back and bend both knees. Bring your feet close to your hips. Keep your feet hip-width apart and heels on the floor. Place your hands by your sides with your palms facing down.
→   Breathe in and push your hands into the floor. Slowly lift your hips up towards the ceiling. Reach with your hands towards your ankles and bring your chest towards your chin. Your chin should be facing towards the ceiling. Keep pushing your knees slightly towards each other and keep your thighs active. Breathe deeply into your belly. Keep lifting your pelvis upwards and back towards your head.
→   Inhale and exhale evenly for 10 deep breaths, or about a minute.

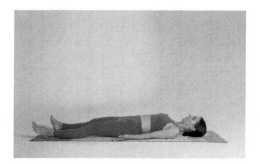

4. CORPSE POSE
O   This is the final relaxation pose. It helps to calm the nervous system and reduces stress.
→   Stay in this pose for as long as you have time, at least a couple minutes.
→   Lie on your back with your legs separated and with your arms by your sides, palms facing up. Close your eyes and breathe naturally. Relax all parts of your body.
→   In this relaxation pose, you can try this breathing technique: Close your eyes and mouth and relax your jaw. Notice the air moving into your nose. Breathe in and out for a count of four. Take a slow exhalation, counting to four. Feel how your chest expands as you inhale and how your belly slightly contracts when you exhale. If you want to go even slower, count to five or six. Repeat five times.

Micro-yoga Relaxation and Breathing Techniques

At the end of the yoga routine, I normally add a short relaxation exercise for the whole body. However, this relaxation exercise can be done on its own any time of the day when you have a space to sit or lie down quietly for five or more minutes. Through relaxation, we work to access the parasympathetic nervous system. This helps us to calm anxiety, reduce physical tension, quiet our mind, and improve sleep.

Relaxation is an important part of the yoga practice. When I am too tired to do anything physical, relaxation is my way to check in with myself, reconnect with my practice and still gain great physical and mental benefits.

Body scan relaxation is a wonderful technique to release tension in the body that we might not even notice that we are experiencing. This type of relaxation technique is founded on the focused attention to all parts of the body in a gradual sequence from feet to head. By bringing focused attention to the whole body, we bring awareness to even subtle bodily sensations like discomfort, tingles, tension, and aches.

The result might not be releasing of all the discomfort completely, but the aim is to get to know the sensations and be able to observe them without movement and without judgement. This way, we will be able to live with them and manage them better.

① FIVE-MINUTE RELAXATION

→ Find a quiet spot and lie down in Corpse Pose. You might want to bring a blanket or a jumper to feel cosy and warm as it increases the relaxation effect. You can also light a scented candle and play gentle instrumental music to create a special atmosphere.

→ When lying down, your arms should be by your sides, palms open towards the sky. Your feet should be in the corners of your yoga mat. Open your chest with a big inhale, then take a long and deep exhale. Bring your chin towards your chest slightly.

→ Take a few deep and slow breaths. Then start breathing from your belly and notice how your belly expands with an inhale and contracts slightly with an exhale. Your eyes are soft; your senses are switched on but relaxed. Your awareness is also open but relaxed. Breathing is natural throughout the entire relaxation.

→ With your eyes closed, gradually bring your awareness towards all of the parts of your body. Do this without moving any part of your body. Just focus your attention on those parts of your body. Notice where your body might hold on to the tension and try to release it with an exhale.

→ Starting with your right foot, try to notice how this body part feels, and whether there is any sensation. Then release any tension with an exhalation. Breathe into any discomfort and see what happens. Visualize the tension leaving your body through your breath. Move on to the next part when you feel ready.

→ Move upwards slowly, with your awareness through your legs, then torso, chest and then through your left leg all the way to your pelvis. Notice how your entire back is grounded on the floor and supported by the ground. Imagine it is melting into the ground below you. Then feel your whole arms, neck and all the parts of your face.

→ Do not judge any feelings or any sensations that arise in your body; just observe and with an exhalation, release and move on to the next part.

→ If any thoughts or noise from the outside world comes to you and disturbs your mind, do not analyse, or hold onto them; just observe them coming and let them go. Give yourself permission to surrender and release any tension or anything no longer serving you.

→ When you are finished scanning all your body parts, you might feel lighter, relaxed, and peaceful. And even if not, stay in this resting pose for a few final breaths.

→ At the end of your relaxation, continue breathing naturally. Your attention should move to your breath, noticing your inhales and exhales. Notice how your breath continues in uninterrupted cycles and brings you what you need for your life. Let exhalation take what does not serve you anymore.

→ When coming out of the Corpse Pose, you can do it mindfully with your eyes closed. Imagine the movement going into the seated position first and slowly repeat the movement with your eyes closed.

→ In a comfortable sitting position, place your hands together in front of your chest. Think about how grateful you are for the moments of relaxation you have given to yourself and thank your body that allowed you to practice. Namaste - bow your head towards your chest!

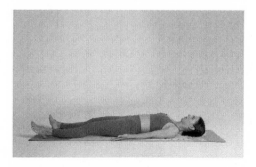

② QUICK CALMING BREATHING TECHNIQUES

These techniques are wonderful for days when you have no energy left or when you feel different challenging emotions. Your task here is to find five minutes to sit still and breathe only according to the instructions of the chosen breathing technique. It might be more challenging at first, but over time, you will see how finding stillness through breathing techniques will be beneficial for your mental health.

I will introduce a few simple breathing techniques that you can do almost anywhere. These techniques can bring wonderful benefits: including stress relief and anxiety, inviting calmness into your life, alertness, and concentration.

Box breathing

This is a wonderful technique to relieve stress and calm the mind. It can also improve concentration and performance. It is called box breathing because all inhales, exhales and pauses between them have the same lengths of time (as the sides of the box). If counting to four is too challenging, it is possible to start counting to three seconds. Someone more accustomed to this breathing technique can start with 5 seconds.

→ Sit with your back supported by a chair. Your eyes should be closed throughout this breathing exercise.
→ Inhale in and count to four slowly.
→ Hold your breath for four counts. Try not to clamp your mouth or nose shut.
→ Then start to exhale slowly for 4 seconds.
→ Hold for four counts, without inhaling.
→ Then repeat the cycle until you feel the calm in your body.

Alternating nostril technique

This breathing technique is a great way to close your yoga routine. It can help to calm your mind. It is also possible to do it separately as part of the relaxation practice. This type of breathing is helpful for infusing the body with oxygen, releasing toxins, reducing stress and anxiety, calming the nervous system, fostering alertness, and helping concentration.

→ For this breathing technique, you will alternate between using your right thumb to close the right nostril and then your right ring finger to close the left nostril. Index and middle finger are touching the place between eyebrows.

→ Close your right nostril with your right thumb. Inhale through your left nostril and pause briefly at the end of the inhale.

→ Next, block your left nostril and release the right nostril; exhale. Take a little pause at the end of an exhale.

→ Keep your left nostril closed and inhale in through your right nostril. Then again, plug your right nostril as you exhale through your left nostril.

→ This completes one round of this breathing technique. The same pattern continues for each additional round: inhale through your left nostril, exhale through your right nostril, inhale through your right nostril, exhale through your left nostril. Repeat for the full five minutes or until you feel a calmness in your body.

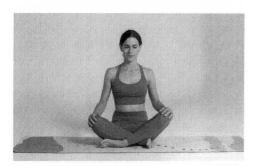

Intuitive Micro-yoga

This is essentially a five-minute free sequence which is completely up to you and your intuition. There are no prescribed yoga poses, no manual; just you, your body and breath. Sometimes it might be a more dynamic sequence, another time it can be gentle yoga stretches or just a relaxation exercise.

Once you have some favourite yoga poses, you can incorporate them into your own sequence. In these five minutes or more, if you have time, you are supposed to just follow your own impulses and let your body and mind provide the answers. I do intuitive Micro-yoga quite often and change my favourite yoga poses so that the routine is a bit different each day. I base this on what my body and mind need and what I feel like doing.

As in every yoga movement, follow your breath, notice how you feel in each pose, be kind to your body, and adjust the pose so that you feel comfortable but still nicely stretched.

After these five minutes where you allow yourself to trust your body and breath, you will feel re-awakened, or relaxed, based on the rhythm your intuition has asked you to follow.

Micro-yoga off the Mat

There are days that are so busy that they do not allow us to even do our quick practice on the mat. We know at the start of the day that most likely we will not fit our yoga practice into our busy schedule. For those times, practising yoga off the mat might be the solution. This way we integrate our yoga practice into our daily rhythm whether we spend it at work or elsewhere.

Yoga can be done almost anywhere, and you do not even need to have a yoga mat with you. A regular short self-care yoga practice brings its results physically and mentally when it fits into your daily life, even when you are off the mat.

In this book we will look at quick sequences any mom can try out in different environments.

① MICRO-YOGA IN THE PARK
② MICRO-YOGA AT THE DESK
③ MICRO-YOGA WHILE COMMUTING
   → MINDFULNESS ON THE GO
   → MICRO-YOGA MOVEMENT DURING A COMMUTE
④ MICRO-YOGA ON THE BED
   → ENERGIZING WAKE-UP ROUTINE ON A BED
   → CALMING BEDTIME ROUTINE ON A BED

① MICRO-YOGA IN THE PARK

When I am outdoors with the kids, I like to do a short exercise to strengthen my body and engage some muscles while watching my kids play. You can try these few yoga asanas when in the park or anywhere outside. It might seem embarrassing at first, but over time you get used to a few looks because nobody minds.

Here is a Micro-yoga sequence for the times when you are outdoors: you can do the whole set for five minutes (and repeat it if you have time) or you can choose just one or two exercises and hold them for a longer time. Again, be kind to yourself and see how you feel in each exercise.

Sequence:
1.   STANDING SIDE BEND
2.   GODDESS POSE
3.   PYRAMID POSE
4.   AIRPLANE POSE
5.   STANDING HALF FORWARD BEND
6.   EAGLE POSE

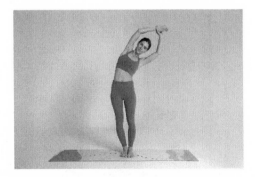

1.   STANDING SIDE BEND
O   Side Bend Pose is wonderful for stretching your back and the sides of your waist. It builds strength in your back, as well as obliques and tones the waist and the side of your body.
→   Begin standing in Mountain Pose. Ground your feet on the floor. Inhale and lift your arms overhead. You can either interlace your fingers with pointer fingers extended or hold your right wrist with your left hand.
→   Bend at your waist to the left while exhaling. Hold for three breaths and then come back to the centre. Lower your arms. Repeat on the other side. Then release your arms to your sides.

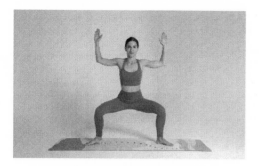

2. GODDESS POSE

O This pose is great for opening your hips, legs, and chest. It strengthens your legs, calves, and knees. It helps to improve your posture and lengthens your spine. It also creates an openness in the pelvis by relaxing muscles.

→ Begin standing in Mountain Pose and step your left leg back about 1 metre away. Pivot your heels to the centre (as if you are on an imaginary yoga mat). Your feet should be parallel to each other. Turn your toes outwards at 45-degrees. You are now in the preparation for a squat.

→ Inhale and bend your knees until your thighs are parallel with the floor. Your knees should not roll in or out and should be lined up with your toes. You should be in a deep squat.

→ Open your chest and draw your shoulder blades back and down and tuck your tailbone.

→ Your spine is straight, and your shoulders are over your hips.

→ Extend your arms overhead and turn your palms toward one another as if you are giving a high five to yourself. Hold the pose for 5 deep breaths. Then come back up from the squat. Lower your arms down and release the pose.

→ It can be quite an intense pose, so you can lessen the squat to keep it easier. Do not bounce your hips up and down and press your heels into the ground.

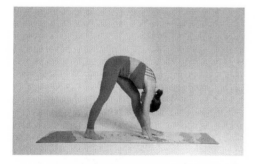

3. PYRAMID POSE

O Pyramid Pose is a great spinal stretch that builds your balance, focus and coordination. It also stretches and strengthens the hamstrings. It works wonderfully to increase their flexibility after running or any daily activities where you bend over.

→ While standing with your feet hip-width apart, step your right leg back about one leg-length, with your right toes pointing toward the upper right corner of your (imaginary) mat. Your stance is like Warrior 1, just shorter.

→ To maintain balance, widen your stance by moving your left foot a little more to the left. Keep your back toes pointing towards the upper right corner.

→ Do not lock your front knee and keep a micro-bend. Turn both hips to face the front (of the imaginary mat). Try to square your hips.

→ Your hands should be on your hips. Fold forward over your front leg, keeping your spine long. Try to bring your fingertips to the ground. If you do not reach it, it is fine, rest your hands on something other than your shin.

→ Your breath should be steady with your legs and abs engaged. Make sure your shoulder blades are drawn away from your ears. Your head should be in line with your spine.

→ Release the pose and slowly straighten your back. Step back into Mountain Pose and repeat on the other side.

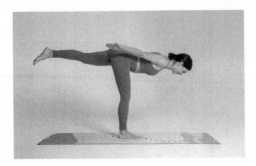

4. AIRPLANE POSE

O This balancing pose creates stability for the whole body and improves your posture, focus and body coordination. This pose really uses all the muscles throughout the core, arms, and legs.

→ Start in the High Lunge position with your right foot forward, and your palms are in the prayer position.

→ Exhale and start lowering your upper body to about a 45-degree angle to the ground.

→ Inhale and start lifting the back foot from the ground but keep the hips square.

Always focus on an unmoving point in front of you. On an exhale, straighten the standing leg. If you feel unstable, keep the front leg slightly bent.

→ Your body and left leg should be parallel with the ground. Lock the knee of the standing leg and engage the right thigh. Keep your lifted foot flexed with toes pointing down.

→ Take five deep breaths in the pose, then bend the front knee, lower the back leg down into the High Lunge and go back to the standing position. Take a few breaths and repeat on the other side.

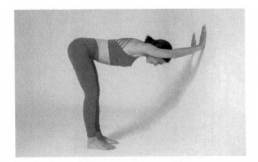

5. STANDING HALF-FORWARD BEND

O Practising this pose is beneficial for stretching your hamstrings, calves, and lengthening the front and back of your torso. It also strengthens your entire spine and improves posture.

→ Start in the Standing Forward Bend. Press your palms or fingertips into the ground beside your feet. With an inhale, straighten your elbows and arch your torso away

from your thighs, finding as much length between your pubic bone and belly button as possible. Place your palms on the tree or something else solid. Bend the knees a little.

→ Look forward and make sure you are not compressing the back of your neck. Your neck should be soft and long. Hold the position for a few breaths. Then release your front body into a forward bend again. Breathe in and out 5 times.

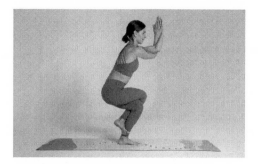

6. EAGLE POSE

O Another pose with enormous benefits
that include building strength in the hamstrings, core, legs to also improving balance
and concentration. It helps stretching upper back, and shoulders, and calves.

→ Start in Mountain Pose. Then bend both knees
slightly, shifting your weight onto your left foot.
Bring your right foot off the ground and cross
your right leg as high up as your left leg as possible. It may be around your ankle or calf.

If this is not possible for you, respect that
and point the foot toward the ground.

→ Cross your right arm under your left,
wrap your forearms/wrists and if possible, bring your palms together.

→ Open your chest and move your shoulder blades down. Stretch up tall
and focus your gaze in front of you,
while taking five deep breaths.

→ Uncross your legs and arms and return to the
Mountain Pose. Repeat on the other side.

After these exercises, stand tall with your arms by your sides.
Close your eyes and notice how you feel; whether there are any
differences you might have experienced in your body.

② MICRO-YOGA AT YOUR DESK

Yoga can also be done at your desk when you sit on a chair at home or at the office. A quick Micro-yoga workout can be done also when sitting outside, just find a stable bench in the park or a playground and have fun with these few exercises. If during this Micro-yoga sequence your attention is concentrated on your breath, it will also increase your mindfulness. These quick exercises can be done every day. It is only necessary to find five minutes for yourself when seated. You can be at the family table, or you can be at work at your desk and still be able to stretch your body and refresh your mind.

When to do it:
→   Before work to stretch a bit and to increase your focus.
→   When you need a mindful break at your desk.
→   When you need to release some stress and ground yourself.
→   After finishing work to release body tension and mental stress.

Sequence:
1.   MOBILIZATIONS OF THE ARMS
2.   HEAD ROLLS
3.   SIDE STRETCH
4.   SPINAL TWISTS
5.   REVERSE PLANK TRICEPS DIPS

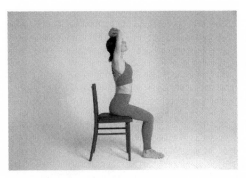

1.   MOBILIZATIONS OF THE ARMS
O   This simple exercise nicely activates your whole spine, creating a nice gentle stretch.
→   Sit on a chair with a long and straight spine. Extend your arms above your head and hold your elbows with your hands.
→   Inhale deeply and extend your arms, without creating any pain.
→   If this feels comfortable, you can take it to a slight back bend. Exhale, come back to the centre and then compensate with a slow forward bend, moving your chin to your chest. Gaze downwards.

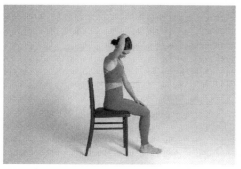 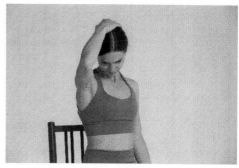

2. HEAD ROTATIONS

O Rotating your head mindfully can relieve your neck of its stiffness and tension, helping to increase the mobility of your neck.

→ After the full head rotations are repeated twice, you can try to draw the infinity sign with your nose. This might gently release some tension in the back of your neck.

→ Inhale and place your right palm on your head. With an exhale, press your head slightly in the direction of your right knee. It should create a nice stretch in the left part of the back of your neck. Stay there for a couple deep breaths. Release the pose, straighten your spine again and repeat on the other side.

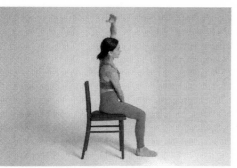

3. SIDE STRETCH

O The benefits of this simple exercise are stretching the side of your torso while engaging the core and the hips. A chair as a prop helps to maintain balance while deepening the stretch.

→ Sit with a straight spine and hold the left armrest with your right hand.

→ Take a deep breath in and extend your left arm up. With an exhale, bend to the right.

→ Your shoulders should be down, away from your ears. Breathe into your chest and feel the stretch across the left side of your torso.

→ Release and repeat on your other side.

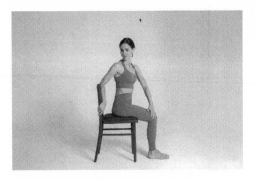

4. SPINAL TWISTS

O A Seated Spinal Twist is beneficial for toning the muscles in your spine, toning your abdomen, and relieving neck and shoulder tension. It also helps with digestion by stimulating the organs in your abdomen.

→ Sit upright and get a hold of the back side of the chair with your right hand. Your left hand should be holding your right knee or the right armrest.

→ Inhale, and with an exhale, rotate to one side slowly and mindfully. Start rotating from your waist with your hips facing forward, then rotate your chest and finish by turning your head.

→ Beware of not pushing through pain. You can place your hand on your chest to help the rotating movement. Your gaze should be behind the chair.

→ Inhale and lengthen your spine. With an exhale, release into a fuller rotation. Breathe in and out 5 times and then return to the starting position. Switch sides.

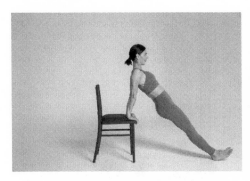
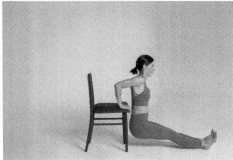

5. REVERSE PLANK TRICEPS DIPS

O Benefits of this exercise are the ability to build your arm and shoulder strength. It is also a great way to increase your upper body strength.

→ Sit on the edge of the chair and grip the edge next to your hips. Your fingers should be pointed at your feet. Your legs are extended, your feet should be about hip width apart with the heels touching the ground. Look straight ahead with your chin up.

→ Press into your palms to lift your body and slide forward just far enough so that your glutes are slightly away from the edge of the chair.

→ Lower yourself until your elbows are bent between 45 and 90 degrees.

→ Slowly push yourself back up to the starting position and repeat 5 times.

→ Breathe slowly throughout the entire movement. At the end, release the pose and come back to the starting position.

③ MICRO-YOGA ON YOUR COMMUTE

Commuting is a part of the daily routine for a lot of moms, and it can be a stressful part of the day. Being in a hurry, getting kids ready to go in the morning and then being stuck in a traffic jam can certainly take a toll on our peace of mind. It does not have to be that way. Easy yoga poses and breathing techniques can make commuting more bearable. They can help the physical posture and calm the mind.

Here, I will introduce a quick series of yoga practices that can be done next time you are stuck in traffic while commuting to your work or running errands for your family. Yoga movements can be done anywhere on a daily commute when it is not a distraction. That means that in a public transport it can be done anytime. In a car, it needs to be done before the drive or when the car is at a complete stop. Other practices inspired by yoga can be done anytime during a commute.

One of the best ways to start a commute is to set an intention. Take a deep breath in and set an intention in your mind. Form a positive statement in your mind as if the commute has already happened. I have a safe and pleasant journey to work. I am calm and ready for the day. Inhale and exhale slowly as this intention sinks in and visualize how you travel with no rush. Then you can begin your commute.

The easiest technique to incorporate into your daily commute is pranayama or yogic breathing. It is invisible, has incredible benefits and can be performed anywhere. Deep yogic breathing helps to build mindfulness of the present moment, decrease the stress response of the rush-hour, helps to slow the heart rate, and increase focus. All these breathing techniques have calming effects to mitigate anxiety and tension.

Equal Breathing

Another technique that is similar to the Box Breathing introduced earlier is the Equal Breathing technique. For this technique, you inhale and exhale through your nose for the same number of counts. You can start with inhaling for four counts and exhaling for four counts. Once your lung capacity expands, you can increase this to five or six counts.

Letting Go

The difference in this breathing technique is that the exhale is through the mouth, making an audible huffing sound, letting go of any tension, while inhaling for four counts. Visualization of letting go of any worries and stress works best. Repeat three times.

Mindful Travel

This might be the easiest technique when you are just being an observer to the world around you. Notice your surroundings, with an open mind, and without judgement observing the world around you. Notice the colours, the sounds, and the smells around you. Be aware of the touch of the seat you might be sitting on or how you hold the handle. Notice if you feel any taste of the coffee or meal you have eaten. And lastly, notice how your breath flows in and out of your body. Notice the expansion of your chest and belly while inhaling and slight contractions when exhaling. If any distracting thoughts or sensations arise, let them go with a mindful exhale.

For the onward journey:
1. SHOULDER ROLLS
2. NECK RELEASE
3. SPINAL SEATED TWIST
4. HIP OPENER

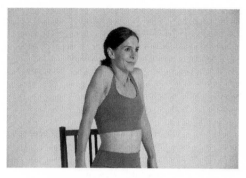 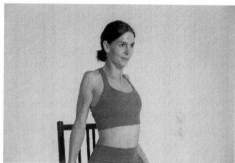

1. SHOULDER ROLLS
O This is a wonderful quick way how to awaken the shoulder area and release any tension.
→ Drop your shoulders down and start slowly rolling them to the rhythm of your breath.
→ Repeat five times both ways - both clockwise and anti-clockwise.

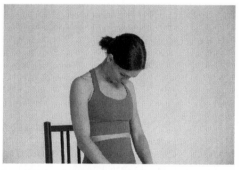 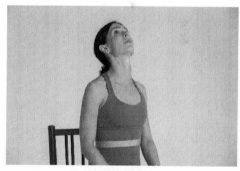

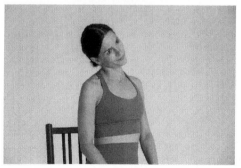 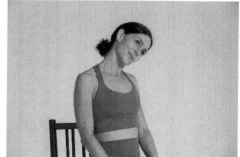

2. NECK RELEASE
O This is a quick exercise to release any tension and discomfort in your neck.
→ Breathe in and look up, point your chin towards the sky or roof of your vehicle.

Exhale and look down. Bring your chin close to your chest. Repeat five times.
→ Inhale, look towards the right, exhale, and come to the centre. Breathe in and turn to the left. Repeat five times.

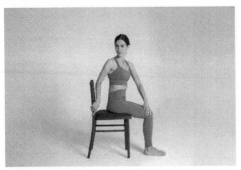

3. SPINAL TWIST
O   This seated twist helps stretch the sides of your spine and increases the range of motion of the muscles around the spine.
→   Sit with your feet grounded firmly on the floor. Place your left hand on your right knee and your right hand behind the pelvis, left thigh, or grab a piece of your clothes.
→   Inhale deeply to lengthen through the spine and the chest. Exhale and slowly start to twist. Take 5 deep breaths and switch sides.

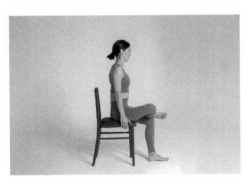

4. HIP OPENER
O   This exercise helps with reducing the stiffness at the hips and loosens up the joints.
→   Sit tall and place your feet hip-distance apart. Ground your feet on the floor and feel it beneath them. Cross your right leg over your left at a 90-degree angle. Keep your right foot flexed to protect the knee.
→   Maintain a straight spine, while distributing the weight equally between your sit bones. Feel the stretch in your thigh and exhale into the stretch. Take 5 deep breaths, then change legs and repeat on the other side.

④ MICRO-YOGA ON THE BED

Sometimes we feel like we do not even want to move a muscle and wish to stay in bed all day. This short and easy sequence is ideal for those days when we do not have any motivation to do an intense workout, but we feel our body needs a little stretch. It even requires staying in bed where all these exercises can be done. Thus, there is no excuse not to find five minutes for lying in the bed in the morning or finishing the day with a fantastic little routine to prepare you for a peaceful doze off.

→ ENERGIZING WAKE-UP ROUTINE ON A BED

This is a wonderful short routine to help you roll out of bed energized. It warms up the entire body and wakes up your mind. To avoid feeling sluggish all day, it is possible to transform your morning in bed by adding these simple yoga stretches as the first thing you do once you open your eyes. Do not wait until you check social media as this might leave no time and motivation for this simple stretch. Of course, if you need to nurse your baby or wake up an older kid, do what is necessary and if you have time for a little lie in later, while your partner looks after the children, you can return to bed for a simple routine. Again, listen and be gentle to your body throughout the whole sequence. If you feel any discomfort, readjust the pose.

Sequence:
1.   WAKE-UP FULL BODY STRETCH
2.   SEATED CAT COW
3.   CAMEL POSE
4.   SEATED FORWARD FOLD
5.   COBRA POSE
6.   HALF LORD OF THE FISHES POSE

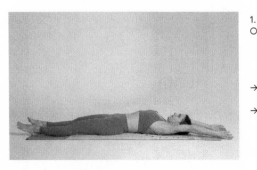

1.   WAKE UP FULL BODY STRETCH
O   Many of us tend to sleep on our sides in a fetal position, which is calming for sleeping and rest. This stretch brings an energy to the whole body, stretching the spine and hips, helping you to wake up.
→   Lie on your back and start wiggling your fingers and toes gently.
→   Extend your arms over your head and notice the stretch throughout your entire body. Point your feet and flex your toes to bring your awareness back to your body. Stay in this position for 5 breaths.

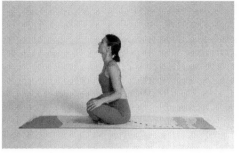 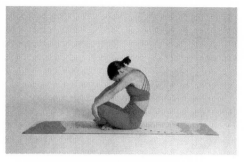

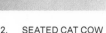

2. SEATED CAT COW

O   This seated pose is a beautiful coordination between breath and movement, facilitating conscious breathing and promoting clarity of mind. It also opens your chest and lungs. It creates more flexibility in the spine and reduces lower back pain and shoulder tension.

→   Place your palms on your knees and sit up tall.

→   To go into a Cat Pose, take a deep inhale in and roll your shoulders forward as you exhale. Tuck your chin in towards your chest. Round your back and pull your belly in.

→   Take a deep breath in and roll your shoulders back, moving your spine in towards your chest while you gaze upwards.

→   Take 5 deep breaths, moving with the rhythm of your breath.

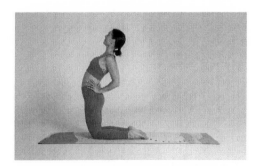

3. CAMEL POSE

O   This backbend stretches the whole front of your body and improves mobility of your spine. Beware of this pose and be very gentle if you have had an injury or a chronic issue with your knees, back, neck or shoulders.

→   Kneel with a straight spine and hips over your knees. Fold a blanket under your knees if they are sensitive.

→   Bring your hands to your lower back with your fingers facing upward and squeeze your elbows towards each other, pointing back.

→   With an exhale, gently arch your back into a backbend. Lift your chin up slightly and open your chest.

→   Bring your hips forward so that they stay over your knees. If it feels good, let your head come back, opening your throat. If it is not comfortable, you can keep the chin tucked instead.

→   Take 5 deep belly breaths. In this position go only as far into the backbend as it is comfortable, never into the pain.

→   Make sure you keep your thighs upright, staying vertical and do not slant backwards.

→   Release by bringing your body slowly into the upright kneeling position.

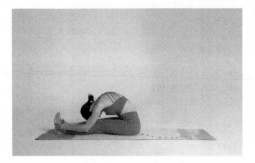

4. SEATED FORWARD FOLD

O Seated Forward Bend is a brilliant stretch for the whole back of your body, from your calves to your hamstrings and your whole spine. It also helps open your hips; it is excellent for tight hamstrings.

→ Sit with extended straight legs. Bring your arms up over your head and reach them towards the ceiling.

→ As you exhale, begin to bend forward, hinging at your hips.

→ On each inhale, lengthen your spine a bit longer. You can come a bit out of your forward fold to do this.

→ On each exhale, go deeper into your forward bend. Imagine your belly coming to rest on your thighs, rather than your nose coming to your knees. This will help you keep your spine long.

→ Your neck is the extension of your spine, neither cranking it to look up nor letting it go completely.

→ When you have come to your full bend with a long spine, let it round forward. Grab your ankles or shins, whichever you can reach. Your feet should be flexed strongly throughout. Take 5 deep breaths with a rounded spine.

→ To release, come back slowly into the upright seated position.

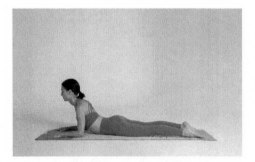

5. SPHINX POSE

O This is a wonderful pose that strengthens your back muscles, stabilizes your shoulders, and stretches your abdomen.

→ Lie on your stomach and place your elbows under your shoulders. Elbows are pointing back, not to your sides. Your forearms and palms should be flat on the floor.

→ Inhale and engage your ab muscles, lifting your chest and shoulders off the ground. Bring your shoulders back away from your neck. Focus on extending through your upper back, instead of contracting your lower back.

→ Stay in this pose for 5 deep breaths. Make sure that your spine feels lengthened, instead of compressed. You can bring your elbows forward if you wish to reduce intensity. Keep your hips on the bed and your neck relaxed.

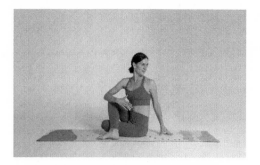

6. HALF LORD OF THE FISHES POSE

O This twist invites energy to your spine and lower abs, stimulating digestion and alleviating constipation, while improving postural awareness. It also stretches around your back, thighs, and gluteus.

→ Sit upright with your straight legs extended in front of you while keeping your feet together.

→ Bend your left leg and place the heel of your left foot beside your right hip. If this is not comfortable for your hips or knee, keep your left leg straight.

→ Move your right leg over your left knee.

→ Place your right hand on your right knee and your left hand behind your back.

→ Start rotating from your waist, shoulders, and neck to the left and look over your left shoulder. Keep your spine long and straight.

→ Alternatively, you can rotate to the right (placing the left hand on the right knee). Try it both ways to see how it feels for you and notice the difference.

→ Hold the pose for 5 long inhales and exhales.

→ Exhale and release the hand behind your back first. Next release your waist, then chest, then neck. Finally, sit up straight.

→ Repeat on your other side. Then come back to the front and relax.

At the end of this sequence, you can put your hands in front of your chest, remember your intention for the day and say a little gratitude in your mind. Now you are ready to seize the day.

→ CALMING BEDTIME ROUTINE ON A BED

Slow and gentle yoga can be the perfect way to relax your muscles and your mind at the end of a long day. This routine can allow you to unwind, release the stress of the day, and prepare your body and mind for a restful night.

If the time allows, you can spend more time in the poses so that they can have a more relaxing effect. However, you can feel the benefits even in five minutes, and you will be ready for a peaceful sleep.

Sequence:
1. FOLDED BUTTERFLY POSE
2. SEATED WINDING DOWN TWIST
3. HERO OR RECLINED HERO POSE
4. HAPPY BABY POSE
5. RECLINING BOUND ANGLE POSE
6. SUPPORTED CHILD'S POSE

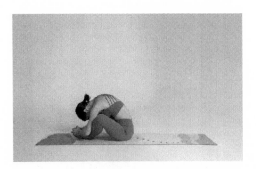

1. FOLDED BUTTERFLY POSE
O This pose is a great hip opener and stretch for the lower back. It is fantastic for those with tight hips and lower back pain, which is usual after a long day at the desk.
→ In a comfortable seated position bring the soles of your feet together in front of you.
→ Find what feels good for your feet; to have them as near, or far away from your pelvis.

Sit on a pillow or support your knees on either side with pillows if you need to.
→ Take a deep breath in and lengthen your spine. Then gently fold forwards, curving your spine and neck to bring your forehead towards your feet.
→ Stay in this pose for 5 deep breaths.

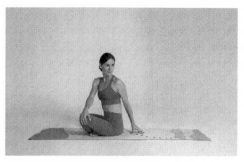

2. SEATED WINDING DOWN TWIST
○ This relaxing yoga pose promotes good digestion and spinal mobility. Twisting helps to tone the abdomen, massage internal organs and can alleviate lower back pain.
→ Sit cross-legged with a straight spine.
→ Put your right hand on your left knee and your left hand on the bed behind you.
→ Exhale as you start to rotate your torso slowly to the left, allowing your eyes and head to follow.
→ Continue lifting through your spine with each inhale and rotate more with each exhale.
→ Stay in the twist for 5 deep breaths, then return to centre, release the pose and switch sides.

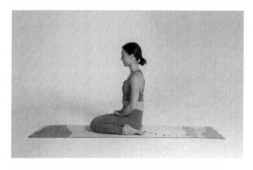

3. HERO POSE/RECLINED HERO POSE
○ Hero Pose is a brilliant pose for stretching the quadriceps and ankles, as well as helping to build flexibility in those areas. The spinal alignment in Hero Pose attacks the slouching posture and allows for better breathing.
→ Put a pillow under your sit bones to make it more comfortable. You may also want padding under your ankles if you feel any discomfort.
→ Keep your knees together in this pose as you spread your feet apart so that

you can sit between your feet. Do not sit on your feet, but between them, so that the toes are tucked under.
→ Your feet should point straight back, turning neither inwards nor outwards.
→ Slide your shoulders away from your ears. Rest your hands in your lap.
→ If possible, remain in this pose for 5 deep breaths with your eyes closed.
→ Release by pressing your palms into the floor and lifting your butt. Cross your ankles beneath your body and extend your legs in front of you.

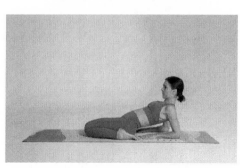

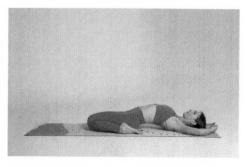

○ You can also try a more advanced reclined variation if you feel comfortable by leaning on your hands, then on your forearms and elbows. You can stay on your forearms for five deep breaths. Alternatively, you can continue to release your lower back and the entire back on the mat or on a support blanket.

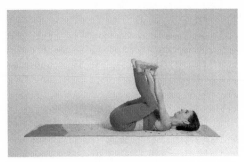

4. HAPPY BABY POSE

O   This pose can improve flexibility and reduce lower back pain, thanks to being able to stretch the inner thighs, hamstrings, and groin. This releases the hips and back and realigns the spine. It also has a wonderful calming effect, reducing stress and anxiety.

→   Lay down on your back and bring your knees to your chest.

→   Bend your knees towards your chest at a 90-degree angle, with the soles of your feet facing towards the ceiling.

→   Hold the inside or outside of your feet. Spread your knees apart, shifting them towards your armpits.

→   Inhale deeply and allow your body to rock side to side slowly.

→   Remain in this pose for 5 deep breaths.

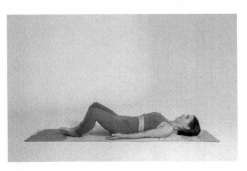

5. RECLINING BOUND ANGLE POSE

O   This restorative pose stretches the thighs, groins, hips, and relaxes the internal organs. It also stimulates the heart and improves the blood circulation. This pose is wonderful for relaxing pregnant women, as well as relieving symptoms during PMS. At bedtime, it is supposed to have great effect on alleviating insomnia.

→   Lay down on your back, with your knees bent. Your arms stay beside you on the bed.

→   Bring the soles of your feet together and focus on letting your knees fall open, do not force them down.

→   If you feel any discomfort in your hips, support your legs with pillows under each knee.

→   Stay in this pose for 5 breaths, then extend your legs out.

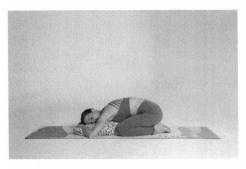

6. SUPPORTED CHILD'S POSE

O   This is a perfect pose to end the sequence – it stretches your hips and back as well as relaxes the central nervous system. Of course, there is always a yogic choice and if you prefer, you can choose a simple lying Corpse Pose to end this routine.

→   Take a bigger pillow and sit on one end, with your thighs extended to your sides and your sit bones against your heels.

→   Gently fold forward to rest on the pillow, with your head turned to one side, keeping your sit bones and heels together if possible. If not, put a blanket or pillow between them.

→   Rest on the pillow, trying to let go of any distracting thoughts.

→   Stay here for 10 breaths, then repeat with your head facing the opposite direction. Do not worry if you doze off in this pose.

After this sequence you should feel relaxed and ready to tuck into the duvet and drift off to sleep.

These are all the routines off the mat that I wanted to cover in this book. However, you can perhaps think of other places where you can do some simple yoga movements. It would be great for your body and mind if you can incorporate quick Micro-yoga as much into your days as possible.

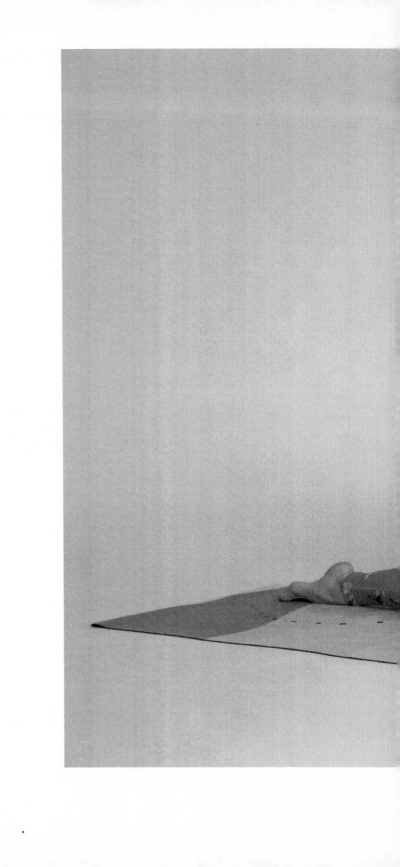

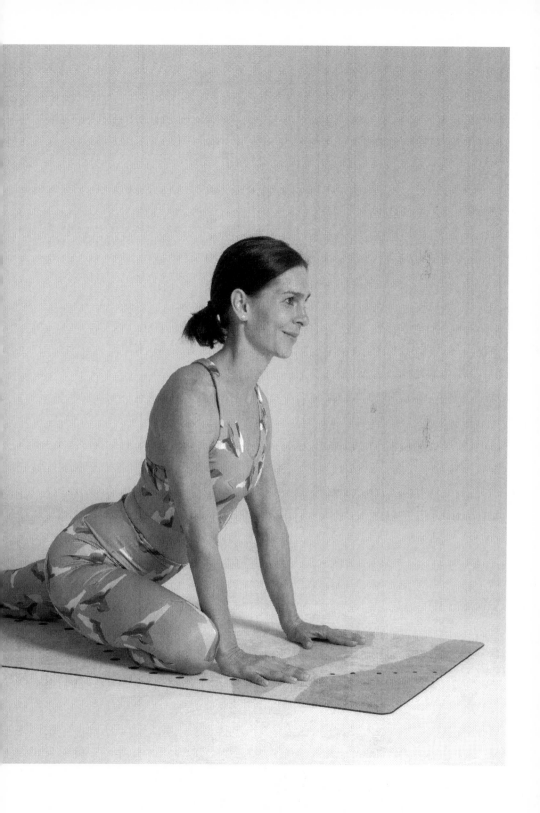

Conclusion

It is March 2021 and one year has passed since the first lockdown. We are again in the same situation with my whole family still at home. Now it is a toddler, pre-schooler, my husband, and me. We are looking after the kids, working from home, and trying to cope with all the responsibilities in this unpredictable world. Something has changed though. Every day without an exception, I do my yoga practice for at least five minutes. It is my commitment to myself and my self-care. Sometimes it is just lying down to do some gentle poses, another day it is a longer dynamic practice. Sometimes it is yoga in the park with my kids. My practice is a work-in-progress.

I am still a work-in-progress. No, I am not a mom full-of-zen and a peaceful partner all the time. I still get overwhelmed, irritated, and tired. In those times, I try to be compassionate towards myself and I understand that I need to put my wellbeing first to recharge myself. Now I understand that to be full-of-energy and to handle all the changes and the frenetic pace of life, I need to prioritize caring for my body and mind. And this is what Micro-yoga has taught me.

Micro-yoga is based on two main arguments. First is that micro-routines are an achievable everyday win, and thus ideal for busy people who want to start a new self-care ritual but are limited with time. Micro-yoga practices can be built into our daily rhythm no matter how busy we are. Prioritizing small self-care activities daily rather than lavish interventions occasionally has a much greater effect.

The second argument is that yoga is great for both the body as well as the mind. Yoga has proven to bring multiple physical and mental benefits. This way the regular practice improves the physical and mental health. Therefore, it should be an essential part of any mom's personal care.

In this book, I have provided you with the tools to equip you to get started with Micro-yoga practice. Micro-yoga presented in this book is available for all moms with any level of fitness and flexibility and is suitable for yoga beginners. After explaining the need for self-care for moms and the benefits yoga brings, I have looked at some essential foundations such as the time, the space, and the support you need to have in place for your practice to begin and be consistent. I have provided you with the key principles of any yoga practice and a quick overview of the main yoga styles that are influential for the routines mentioned in this book.

I have divided the Micro-yoga practices into the post-natal practices suitable for new moms and the dynamic and calming quick routines for all moms. By now, you might have learned the recommended first dynamic and calming Micro-yoga routines. Later, you could have chosen any routine depending on your energy level and what practice you need. Once routines on the mat were covered, I have shown you that yoga can be integrated into your life and done almost anywhere off the mat such as at your desk, in the park, during your commute and in bed. If you have read so far, you will have a selection of routines that you can choose from and incorporate into your daily self-care to see the benefits it can bring.

This is not the end. It might be just a discovery of something new about yourself, your body, and your inner world. It is the beginning of a journey. Maybe with yoga, but certainly with your identity, when you slowly become someone who is committed to your personal care, consistently, every day. What you experience on the mat has a ripple effect off the mat. So, do not hesitate. Just take five minutes for your own Micro-yoga ritual every day. You might be surprised where it leads you.

Acknowledgements

I could not have written this book without countless help of my family members, friends, and professionals. First, biggest thanks to my husband Dominik for his encouragement in this whole project. He always supported me in making my dreams come true. Special thanks go to Jana Hetenyiova, Silvia Kancevova, and many other moms who gave me many valuable suggestions that made this book much better. I am also grateful to Audrey Aamot for all her editing work and polishing my writing in English. It has been my privilege to work with Anezka Hruba Ciglerova who has made the world-class book design and layout. Thanks also to those who made the pictures in this book look wonderful: Jana Podrouzkova from Dhaara and Alzbeta Svobodova from One Day shop for borrowing their beautiful yoga mat and clothes, as well as photographer Tereza Havlinkova. Finally, I am eternally thankful for my two little boys Sam and David who inspired me to write this book and bring me joy and love every day.

About the Author

Zuzana is a certified yoga teacher specializing in hatha, vinyasa flow, and pregnancy yoga. Outside of yoga, she is a training and talent development professional who has worked in different industries. She lives in Prague with her wonderful husband and two beautiful boys.

EMAIL: microyoga.book@gmail.com
INSTAGRAM: zuzka.zee

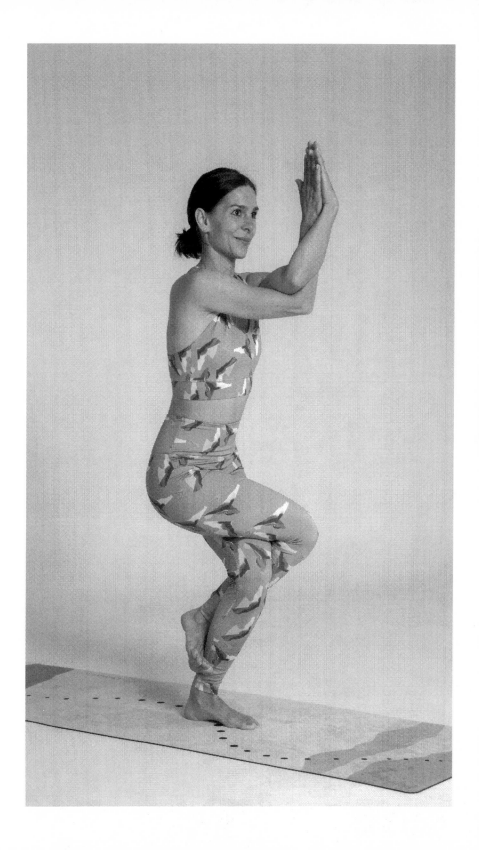

REFERENCES

BMIHealthcare. (2021). What is self care and why is it important? Retrieved from BMIHealthcare: https://www.bmihealthcare.co.uk/health-matters/health-and-wellbeing/what-is-self-care-and-why-is-it-important

Chatterjee, R. (2019). Feel Better in Five. Penguin Life.

Christina M Godfrey, M. B. (2010). The experience of self-care: a systematic review. JBI Libr Syst Rev., 1351-1460.

Clear, J. (2018). Atomic Habits. London: Random House.

Ekhart, E. (2021). The importance of Breath in Yoga. Retrieved from Eckhart Yoga: https://www.ekhartyoga.com/articles/practice/the-importance-of-breath-in-yoga

EkhartYoga. (2021). Finding the balance between effort and ease. Retrieved from Ekhart Yoga: https://www.ekhartyoga.com/articles/anatomy/finding-the-balance-between-effort-and-ease

Kaur, P. P. (2016). Yoga for Happy Moms: Simple techniques for getting your spark back and enjoying parenthood again. Practical Inspiration Publishing.

Kirkova, D. (2014, February 5). Mothers gets just 17 minutes of 'me time' to themselves each day... and STILL take on the lion's share of the chores. Retrieved from Daily Mail: https://www.dailymail.co.uk/femail/article-2552188/The-average-mother-gets-just-17-minutes-time-day.html

Link, R. (2017, August 30). 13 Benefits of Yoga That Are Supported by Science. Retrieved from healthline: https://www.healthline.com/nutrition/13-benefits-of-yoga

Liou, S. (2010, June 26). Meditation and HD. Retrieved from Huntington's Outreach Project for Education at Stanford: https://hopes.stanford.edu/meditation-and-hd/

McKeown, G. (2021). Effortless. London: Ebury Edge.

Norberg, U. (2016). Restorative Yoga : Reduce Stress, Gain Energy, and Find Balance. New York: Skyhorse Publishing.

Outside Interactive Inc. (2021). Restorative Yoga Poses. Retrieved from Yogajournal: https://www.yogajournal.com/poses/types/restorative/

Perel, E., & Miller, M. A. (2020). Esther Perel Blog. Retrieved from Rituals for healthy relationships: https://estherperel.com/blog/rituals-for-healthy-relationships

Schmall, T. (2018, October 3). Parents get way less than an hour per day of 'me time. Retrieved from New York Post: https://nypost.com/2018/10/03/parents-get-way-less-than-an-hour-per-day-of-me-time/

Shortsleeve, C. (2019, November 22). 15 Signs of Caregiver Burnout and How to Recover. Retrieved from Parents: https://www.parents.com/parenting/moms/healthy-mom/signs-of-caregiver-burnout-moms-need-to-know/

Woodyard, C. (2011, July-Dec). Exploring the therapeutic effects of yoga and its ability to increase quality of life. International Journal of Yoga, pp. 49-54.

Yoga Medicine. (2019, May 16). Restorative Yoga: Healing Through Stillness. Retrieved from Yoga Medicine: https://yogamedicine.com/restorative-yoga-healing-through-stillness/

MICRO-YOGA
FOR BUSY MOMS:
Become a calm and fit mom
with quick yoga routines

Published by Zuzana Kosorinova in Prague.
Cover and interior design by Anezka Hruba Ciglerova.
Photos by Tereza Havlinkova.
December 2021: First Edition
ISBN - 978-80-907138-5-7